TIKI BARBER'S
PURE
HARD
WORKOUT

TIKI BARBER

and JOE CARINI with SCOTT HAYS

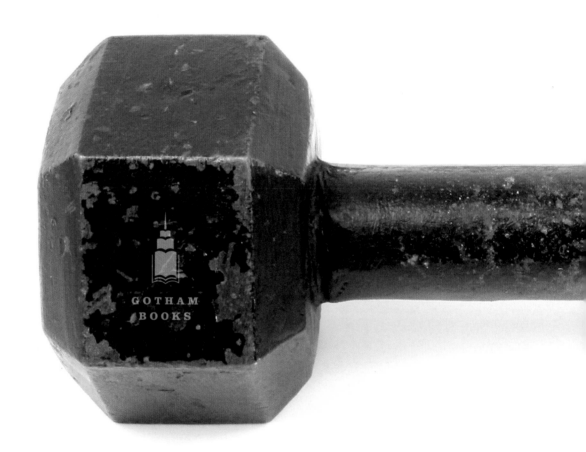

GOTHAM
BOOKS

STOP WASTING TIME and
START BUILDING REAL STRENGTH
and MUSCLE

TIKI BARBER'S

PURE HARD

WORKOUT

GOTHAM BOOKS

Published by Penguin Group (USA) Inc.

375 Hudson Street, New York, New York 10014, U.S.A.

Penguin Group (Canada), 90 Eglinton Avenue East, Suite 700, Toronto, Ontario M4P 2Y3, Canada (a division of Pearson Penguin Canada Inc.); Penguin Books Ltd, 80 Strand, London WC2R 0RL, England; Penguin Ireland, 25 St Stephen's Green, Dublin 2, Ireland (a division of Penguin Books Ltd); Penguin Group (Australia), 250 Camberwell Road, Camberwell, Victoria 3124, Australia (a division of Pearson Australia Group Pty Ltd); Penguin Books India Pvt Ltd, 11 Community Centre, Panchsheel Park, New Delhi – 110 017, India; Penguin Group (NZ), 67 Apollo Drive, Rosedale, North Shore 0632, New Zealand (a division of Pearson New Zealand Ltd); Penguin Books (South Africa) (Pty) Ltd, 24 Sturdee Avenue, Rosebank, Johannesburg 2196, South Africa

Penguin Books Ltd, Registered Offices: 80 Strand, London WC2R 0RL, England

Published by Gotham Books, a member of Penguin Group (USA) Inc.

First printing, November 2008

10 9 8 7 6 5 4 3 2 1

Gotham Books and the skyscraper logo are trademarks of Penguin Group (USA) Inc.

Printed in the United States of America

SET IN SABON AND TRADE GOTHIC

DESIGNED BY JUDITH STAGNITTO ABBATE / ABBATE DESIGN

PHOTOGRAPHS BY MICHAEL TEDESCO

LIBRARY OF CONGRESS CATALOGING-IN-PUBLICATION DATA

Barber, Tiki, 1975–

Tiki Barber's pure hard workout: stop wasting time and start building real strength and muscle / Tiki Barber and Joe Carini with Scott Hays.

p. cm.

ISBN 978-1-592-40396-7 (hardcover)

1. Weight training. 2. Bodybuilding—Training. 3. Physical fitness. I. Carini, Joe. II. Hayes, Scott Robert, 1959– III. Title.

GV545.5.B37 2008

613.7'13—dc22   2008016764

While the author has made every effort to provide accurate telephone numbers and Internet addresses at the time of publication, neither the publisher nor the author assumes any responsibility for errors, or for changes that occur after publication. Further, the publisher does not have any control over and does not assume any responsibility for author or third-party Web sites or their content.

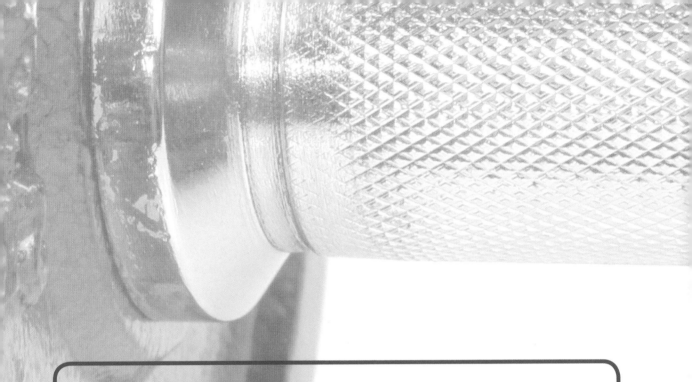

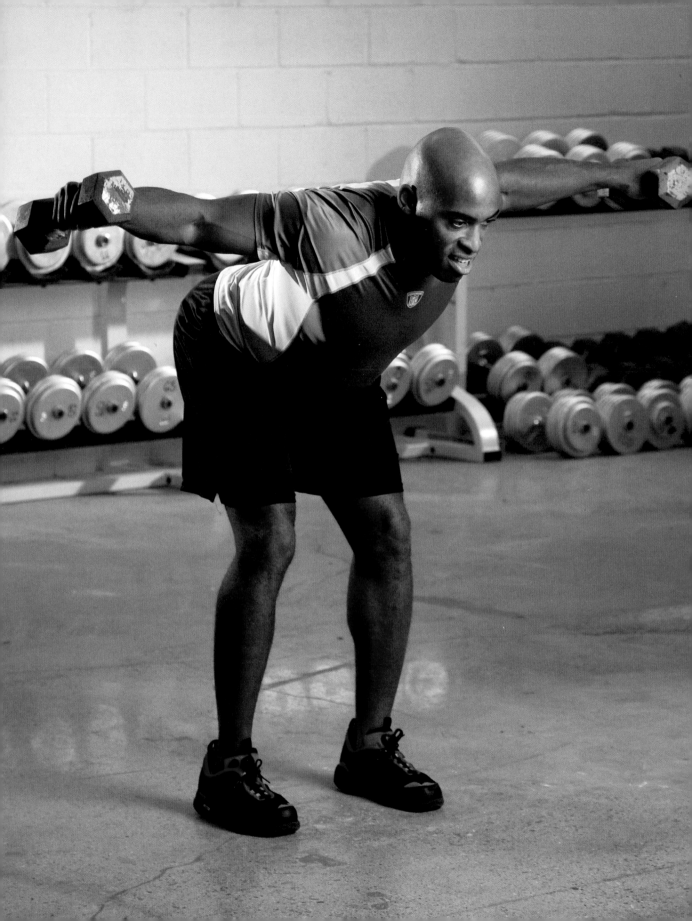

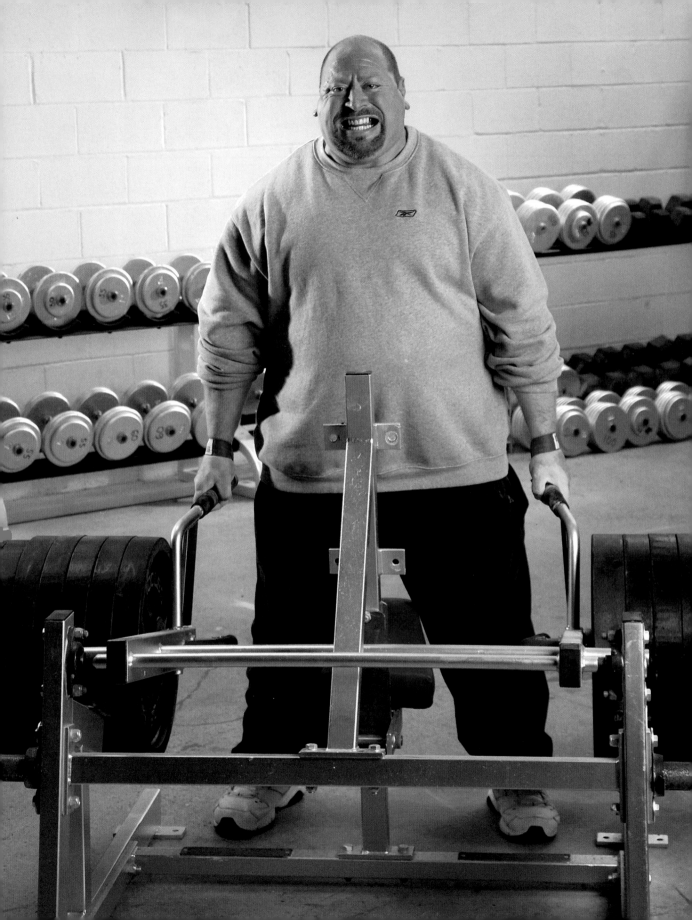

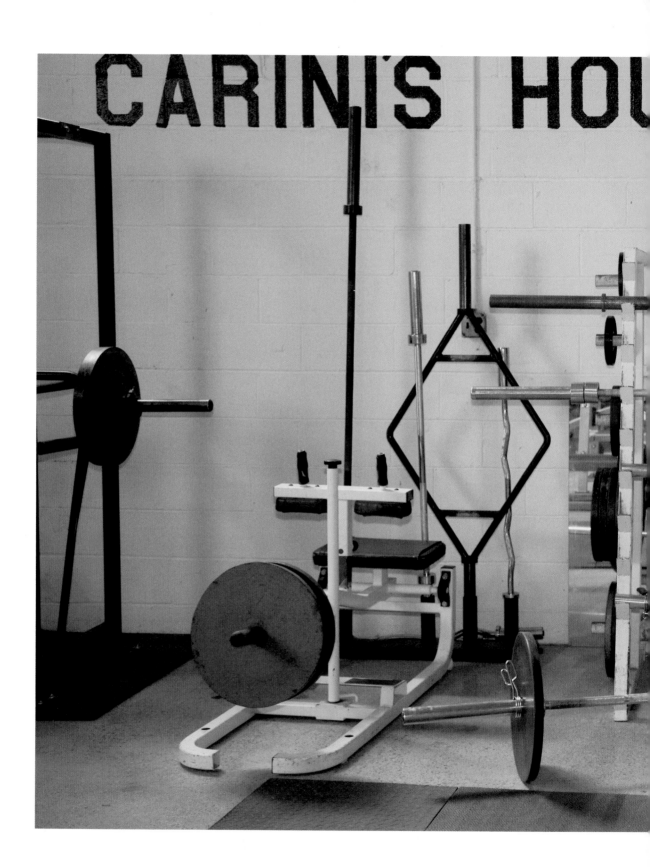

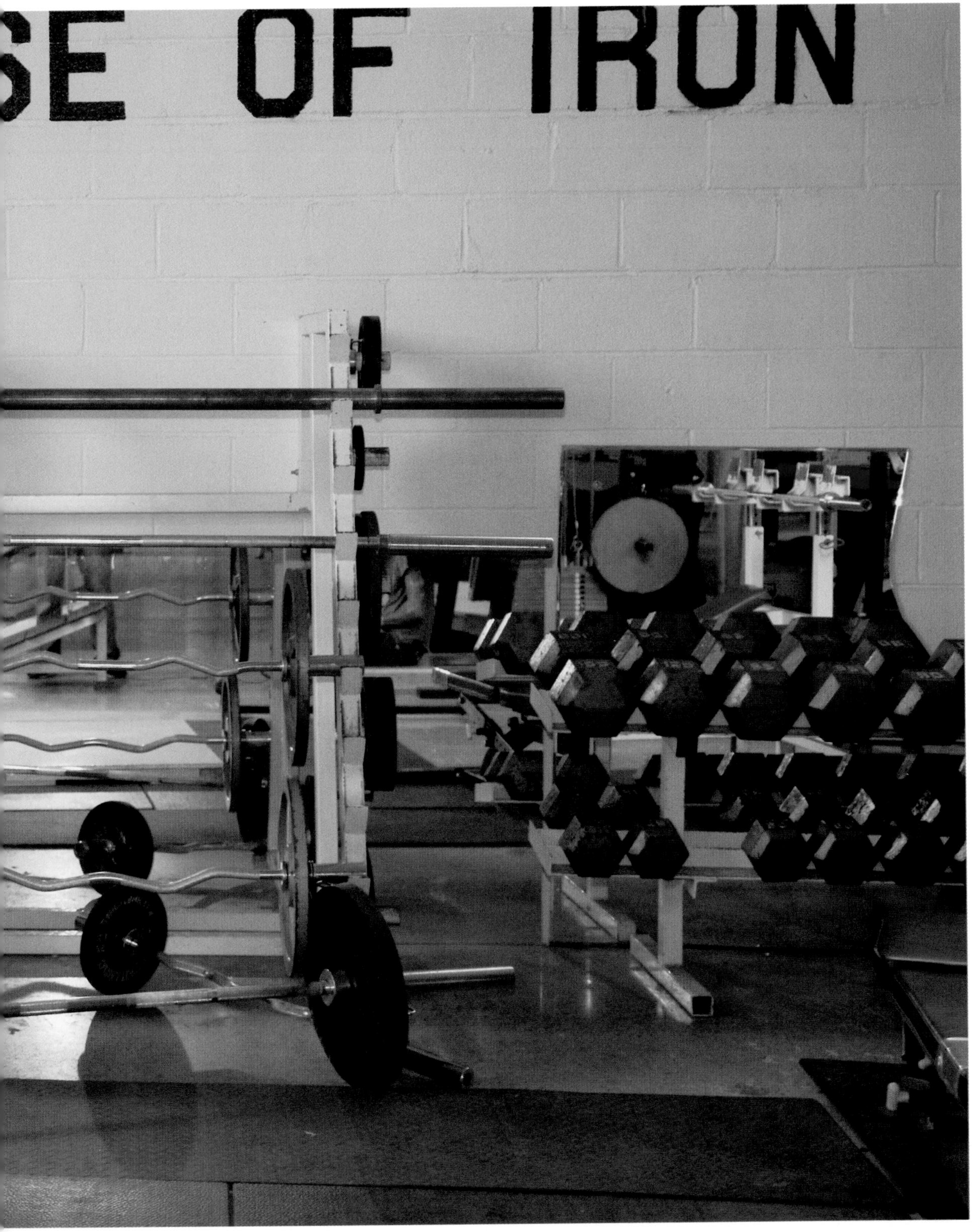
SE OF IRON

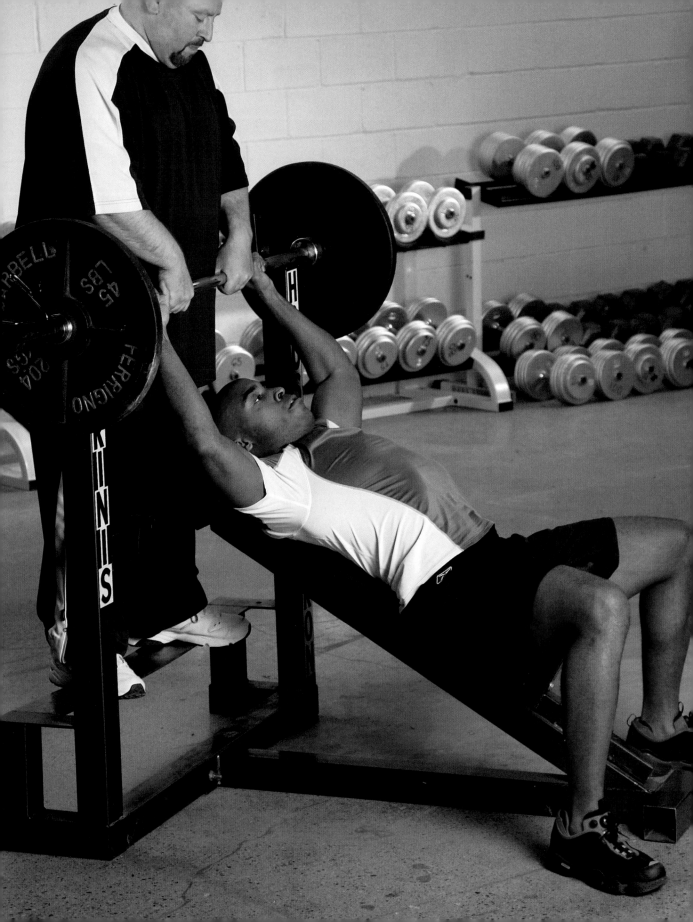

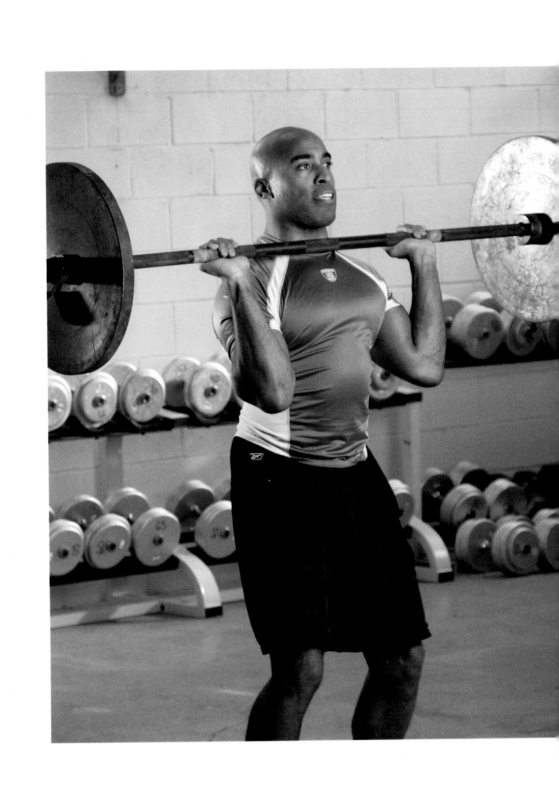

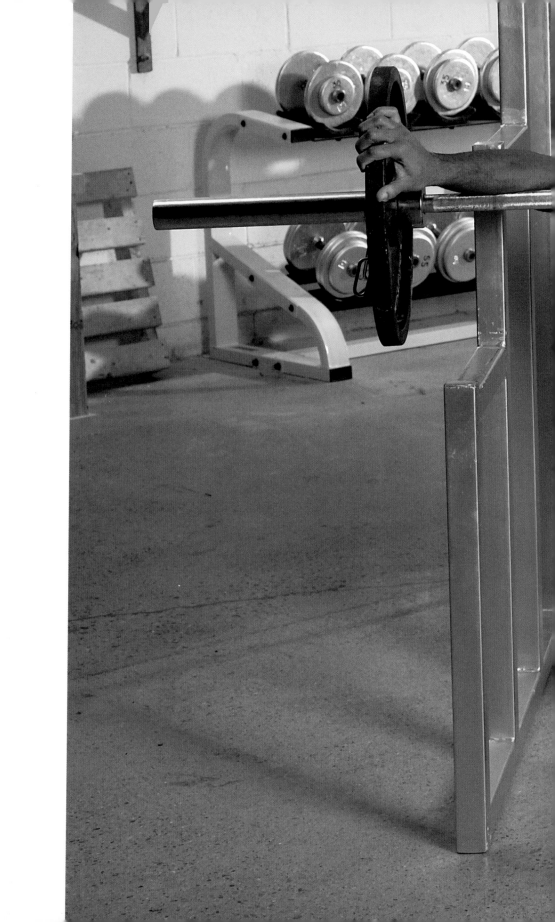

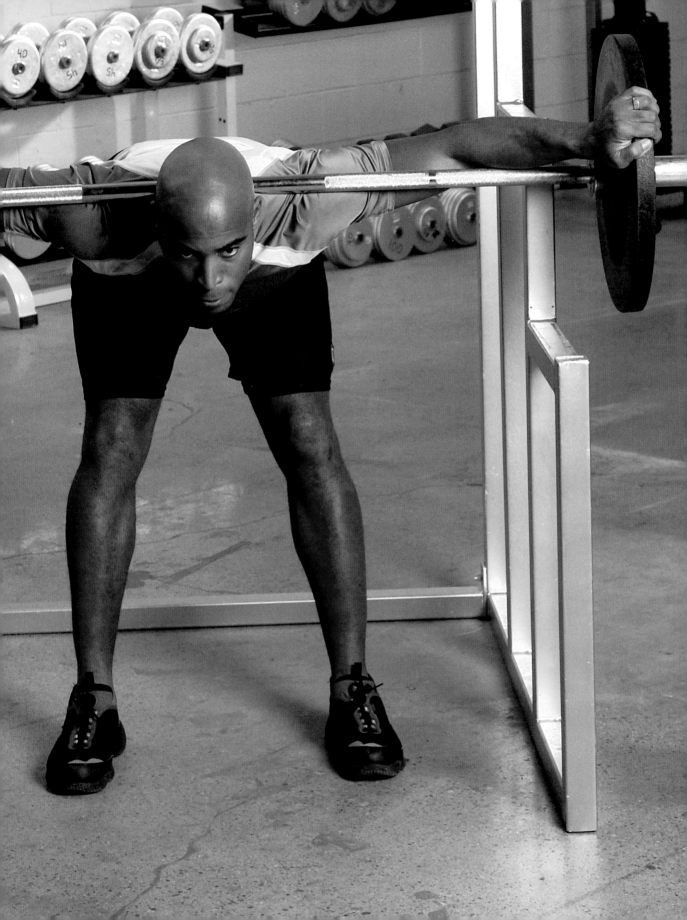

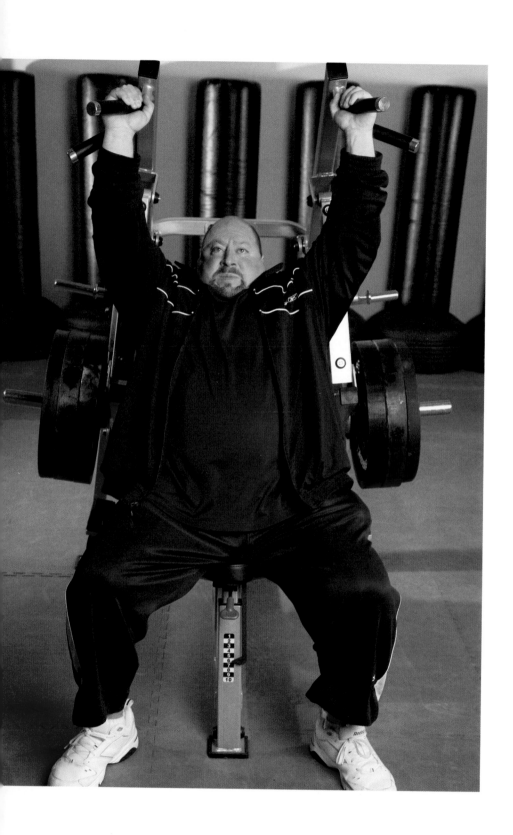
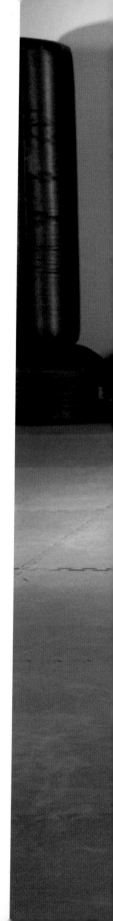

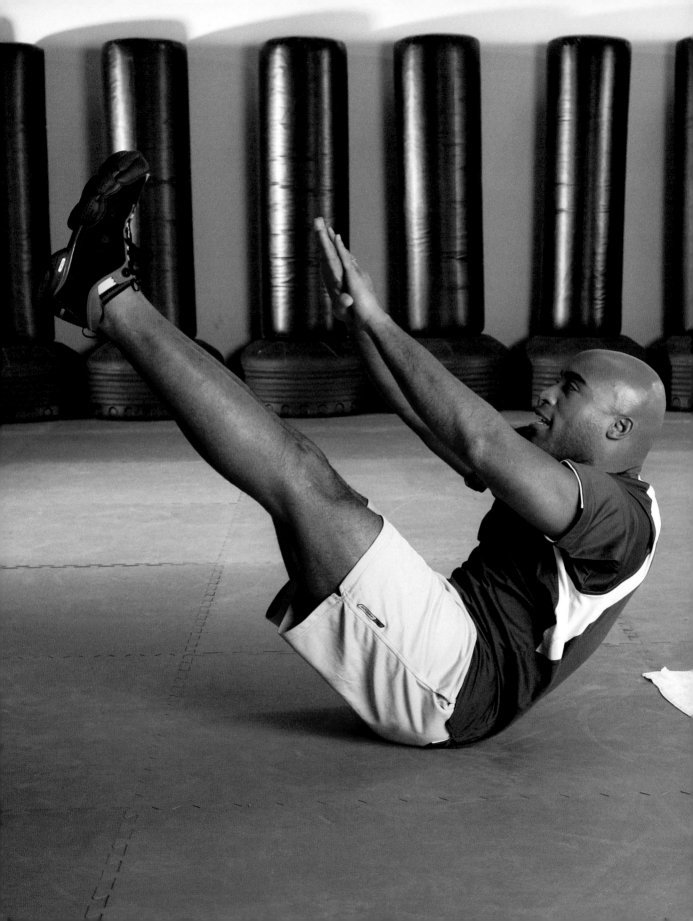

CONTENTS

PART III
DOWN TO PURE HARD WORK

PART IV
THE PROGRAMS

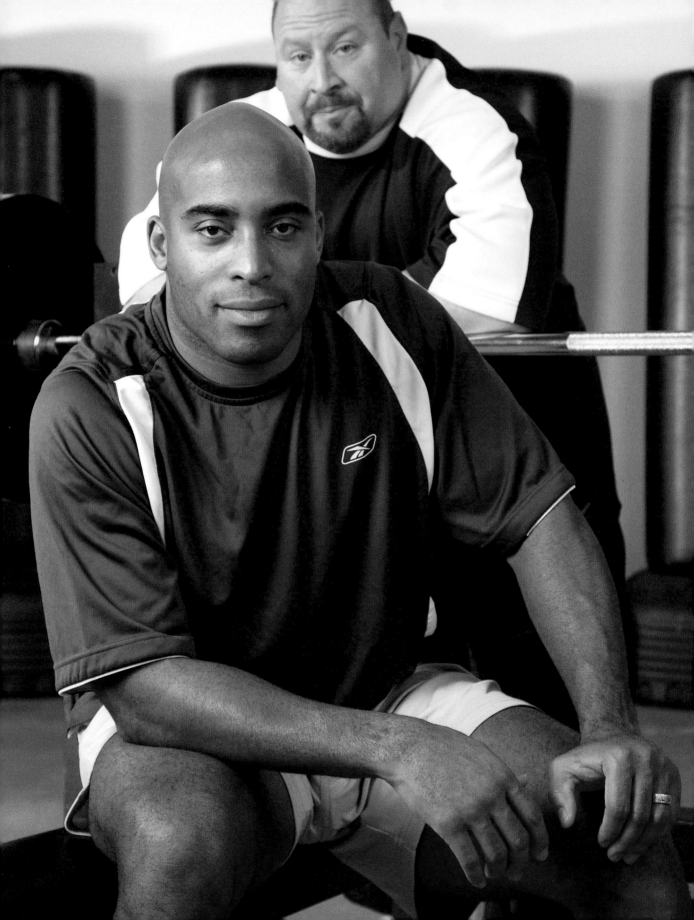

INTRODUCTION

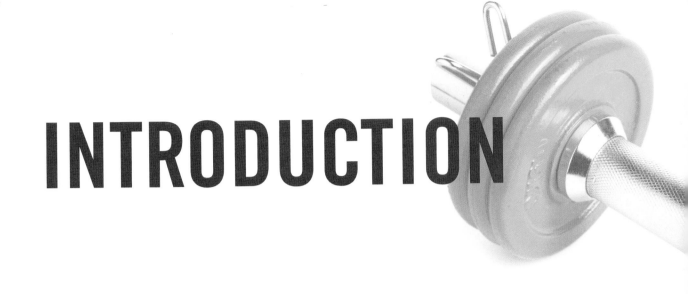

The fitness program you'll find in this book, designed for Tiki Barber by powerlifting specialist Joe Carini, not only flouts conventional wisdom about weight training, sports injuries, and speed; it will also make your body stronger, faster, and more durable. The results Tiki himself achieved with this program have convinced him of its value, and he's pumped about sharing it with the world.

Joe always knew his program would work. But it took the elevation of Tiki Barber from a third-down specialist to one of the most productive running backs in NFL history to prove it to the world.

Tiki came into the league at 5 feet 10 and 190 pounds. His frame was considered too light to absorb the pounding of an every-down player, so Tiki was ticketed as a punt returner and a situational running back when the New York Giants' primary running threat needed a break. In his first three seasons, he carried the ball 136, 52, and 62 times.

Though Tiki was neither the fastest nor the biggest back in the league, he possessed many of the same qualities as the league's best. He had a great feel for the game with remarkable instincts. He could see between defenders and through their holes. He knew when to accelerate, when to slow down, when to set up a block. He could fight through arm tackles and always fell forward for the extra yard. Over the years, he only got smarter. By 2003, he had become the Giants' primary running back and was showing hints of greatness, but his small size and unnerving propensity for fumbling were holding him back.

So in early 2004 he began working with Joe Carini. Under Joe's direction, Tiki got stronger—much stronger. A 190-pounder who could rarely push 300 pounds in the safety squat was transformed into a 200-pounder moving weight into the seven hundreds. Though small in stature, Tiki was able to build a strong back and establish the sort of upper-body strength that combined with his pistonlike legs to allow him to run over defenders until he, remarkably, became an elite back in the NFL and left his mark in the record books.

At the time, Joe trained in one large rectangle, with a track along one wall, a boxing ring next to the finish line, and various punishing machines scattered in the middle. It was in this humble arena that Tiki became the miracle of the locker-room circuit. Joe, a record-breaking powerlifter, pulled Tiki through a regimen that increased speed, strength, and durability. At Joe's direction, Tiki sweated through a tough, at times strange, lineup of exercises, intended first to bulk him up and then to reduce his penchant for dropping the football. Tiki added 18 pounds of rock-hard muscle, and exploded onto the field and then into the record books. He became virtually unstoppable.

"I just felt stronger, and I think confident as well," says Tiki. "You feel like your body has no weaknesses. A lot of what Joe did for me was mental, not necessarily physical—teaching me to fight through tough times. Sometimes he would use a ridiculous amount of weight, and I'd say, 'Joe, this is heavy. This is hard.' He'd say, 'Life's hard.' I never got a break with him."

New Jersey native Joe has been in the game for more than a quarter century, designing exercise programs for both professional and recreational athletes. His own career was littered with various "firsts" (for example, he was the first man in New Jersey to officially squat 800 pounds). Joe was named New Jersey's Strongest Man six years running, and captured three New Jersey state powerlifting championships.

A gifted coach and trainer, Joe translates the technical into technique, and in this book he and Tiki lay out a system that involves low repetitions of extremely heavy weights. The regimen is not for the weak-minded. The priority here is on functional strength built by heavy deadlifting, squats, bench presses, yoke carrying, and, for the most part, few machines. You'll get bigger and look better, but this program isn't for those who only want to look good for the beach. This is for those who want to get fiercely strong. The workout hews to the philosophy that if you're not lifting off the ground, you're not engaging brute strength. No Nautilus machines or Pilates, here. Get ready to meet the Deadlift. Get ready to grunt.

AN UNBEATABLE HILL

Anyone who wants to look forward to a long and healthy life must work to remain physically fit. But fitness is even more important for athletes, employed in professions that require that they push their bodies to the limit. Ultimate success in sports is achieved by those who prepare in three ways—mentally, emotionally, and physically. For the latter, power and durability are key.

I was always a natural athlete. I wrestled in junior high school and I played football and ran track in high school; these two sports followed me to college. I always had the ability and drive to be successful. For a long time, though, I just didn't have the body for it—the body required to be truly great. I also didn't know that outward differentiation begins with inner command.

Growing up, my football idol was Walter Payton. His off-season workouts were legendary, in particular his daily mountain sprints to make himself stronger, better. My fullback at the time, Greg Cornella, introduced me to a mountain trail in Ramapo, New Jersey, about a quarter mile in length and every foot of it straight uphill. He forced me to make that my personal, Payton-like challenge.

Normally this trail is an easy walking path. People go every day just to relax there. To make it fit my bill, to make it hell, we went out at five thirty a.m., in freezing-cold weather, with ice and snow on the ground, and I forced myself to run the whole way. I ran this hill countless times, and I got in great shape, but never once did it get easy. I got better at attacking it, sure, but never was it easy. In a way, that hill took on a life of its own, became a rival, an opponent. It lacked weakness, and it kicked my butt. However, by failing to master The Hill, I grew—especially in mental toughness.

The mental side of the game of football cannot be overemphasized. During my career I often found that sometimes I required genuine, deep, personal thought to truly motivate myself. I had to convince myself that what I was doing was worth it. This is why I believe that my best years in the game came only after I took my off-season conditioning into my own hands. The mental game in sports, and in life, is really the most important one. As I've said, my "Hill" was unbeatable—no matter how much I attempted it, it never got easy.

But unlike The Hill, every player can be beaten. Sometimes it might not be so obvious, but it's there. Sometimes it takes studying film to find it. Often it can't be found except during the course of a game—and then you must be prepared to exploit it. A 95-yard run against the Oakland Raiders on New Year's Eve in 2005 was a good example of that. During my last regular season game against the Washington Redskins, I ran for 234 yards, an NFL record for someone playing in his last regular season. That year, I was the only running back to rush 1,860 yards. I also chalked up more than 500 yards receiving in one season for a total of 2,390 yards, the second-highest in NFL history.

By attacking The Hill, I got better at it, and prepared myself for the winnable battle on the football field. My belief in that was firm, and as a result I developed an inner strength that gave me an edge.

In 2000 I had my first 1,000-yard season. I had arrived, in a way; I'd made myself into a good NFL running back. I still had my weaknesses—most notably, a weakness for fumbling—but I'd made it to the next level, and I had the tools to climb even higher. Still, it would be three more years before I truly joined the elite.

How strong are you in your arms, biceps, and chest? These are areas where a man holds on to the football, and it was only through strengthening these areas that I conquered my tendency to drop the ball.

It all started when Mark Lepselter, my manager, introduced me to a caricature of a man working out of a dump of a gym above a New Jersey Russian community center. But my first workout session with the man running this gym, Joe Carini, let me know that, Hill or no Hill, never had I pushed myself so hard.

Joe's philosophy was simple: life, and specifically football, is about "functional" strength. Anybody can go into a gym and do the same simple, routine exercises over and over again and look decent in the mirror. But will he be functionally strong? Able, say, to carry a linebacker five extra yards for a first down? Or simply lift the living room couch without pulling a muscle?

Everybody needs a catalyst. Joe Carini was mine.

The average "Joe" will get out of this program whatever he puts into it. There is no ceiling. Training and development, physically and mentally, are all in your mind and, in turn, your effort. Follow this program, and you will see significant power and load improvement in your lifts, and added muscle mass as your body learns to grow. You may not be able to shake off a linebacker, but you'll surely have no more problems with that couch.

When people start a weight-training program, they soon realize its many benefits. Often, they begin their program out of shape and weak. Emotionally and psychologically, they often feel inferior. After they start lifting, however, they will experience not only the exhilaration of working out, but also a confidence that

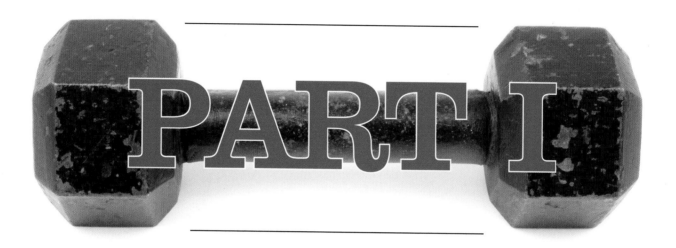

PART I

affects the rest of their lives. To be successful, you must be unwavering in your determination, willpower, and commitment to change. This can be as difficult as the weightlifting itself, but over time the rewards extend outward from your fit body and begin to positively reshape your lifestyle and mind-set. When you have the dedication—work out consistently, never miss a workout, →

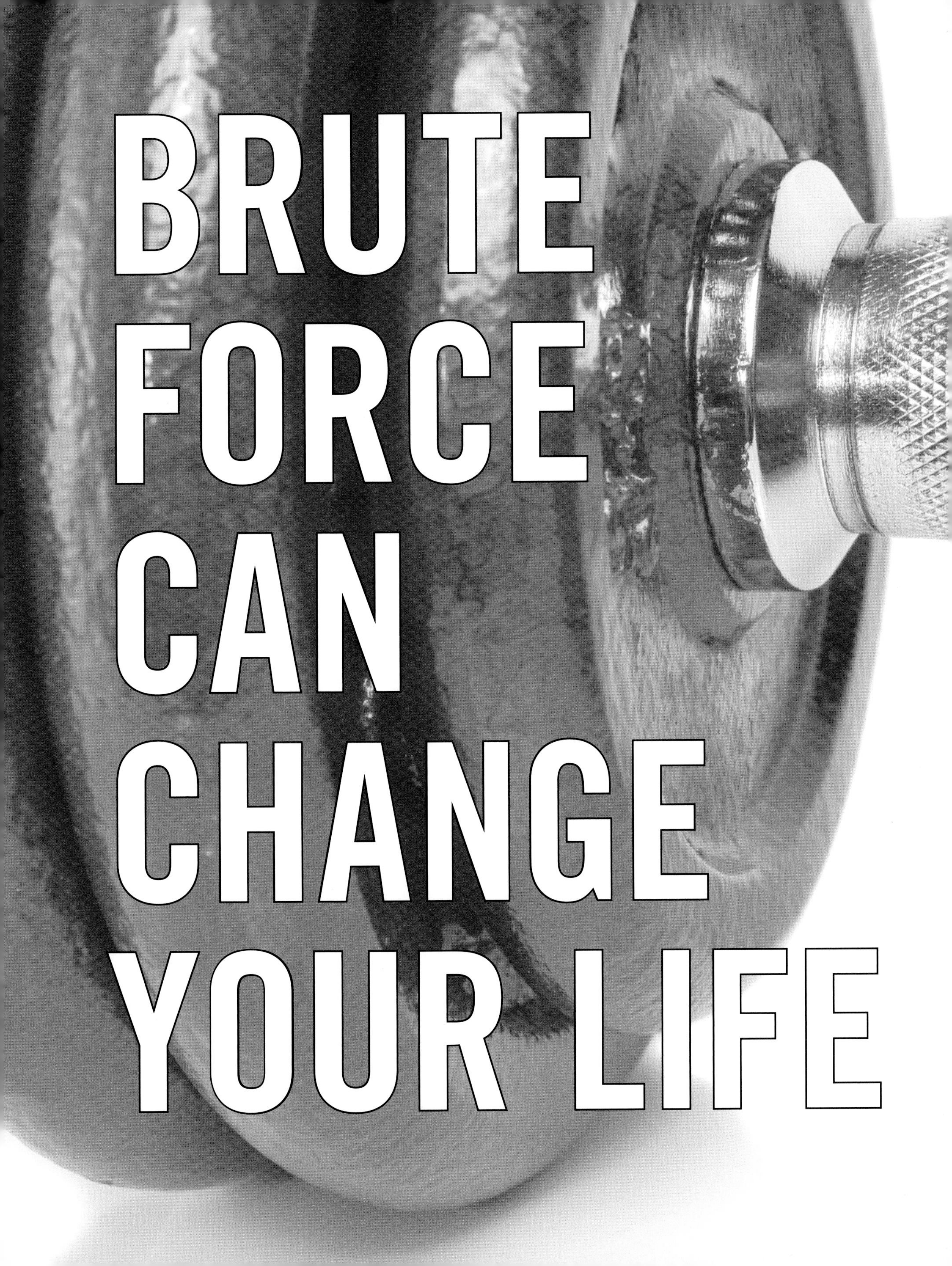
BRUTE
FORCE
CAN
CHANGE
YOUR LIFE

never make excuses for not getting it done—your commitment enhances other aspects of your life. You will, for instance, want to get enough rest to recuperate and prepare for your next workout, and eat right to support your developing muscles.

You just can't consider being an athlete without possessing strength of body and mind. The stronger athlete always wins out to the average player and even to the above-average player. And even those not in sports benefit from lifting because everyone admires the healthy, strong look of the athlete and can appreciate the pure hard work it requires to be in top physical condition. Because the outward muscular training requires mental strength to accomplish, both body and mind develop simultaneously.

Welcome to my work world of pure hard training.

—TIKI BARBER

CHAPTER 1

THE POWERLIFTER AND THE RUNNING BACK

I n a league chock-full of some of the most stellar athletes on the planet, Tiki stood out as one of the hardest working and, pound for pound, arguably the strongest. His transformation has become an accepted miracle. In early 2004 he took his determination and discipline to a new level in a small New Jersey gym during the off-season. He made a commitment to reshape his body *and* his game by hooking up with record-breaking powerlifter Joe Carini, and the

result was the best season of his career to that point.

It's a success story based on trust, experience, persistence, and sweat. A story of two

determined men from very different physical arenas, who together crafted a winning combination of powerlifting techniques. But most of all, it's about how a personal fitness trainer redefined the training objectives of a speedy NFL running back.

In 2005, for example, Tiki put on 18 pounds of pure muscle. When he showed up at training camp that year, his coaches and teammates asked what happened to him. His build resembled that of Hercules, and some of his teammates warned that the league would test him for steroids. The NFL did their mandatory drug tests, and of course Tiki passed every time. Paul Schwartz from the *New York Post*, who'd known Tiki since he was drafted into the NFL, once asked him during an interview if he was on any supplements or drugs. Tiki laughed and summed it up this way: "I'm on pure hard work!"

The workout developed specifically for Tiki included elements of conventional powerlifting as well as strongman exercises. He used sandbags, sled work, and walking with a yoke. Because he was so determined to turn his career around, he eventually succeeded in his goal of dishing out more punishment than he received.

During his first seven years in the league, Tiki rushed for 5,409 yards. During his last three seasons, Tiki rushed for 5,040 yards, an average of 1,680 yards per year. He made Pro Bowl three years running. He also led the NFL in total yards from scrimmage in 2004 and 2005. In addition, Tiki was the first player in NFL history to accumulate 1,800 yards rushing and 500 yards receiving in one season (2005). His career high of 234 rushing yards occurred during his final season in

a game that took place in Washington on December 30, 2006. He earned his record for the most rushing yards of any NFL player during the final game of his career.

The continuous hammering and physical punishment Tiki took without ever missing a game in 2004, 2005, and 2006 are testimony to his strength and power. When Tiki worked out, he didn't just lift weights; he abused them. By using this same method in your training, you will greatly reduce your chances of physical failure in achieving your goals. When you adapt to stress, you compensate for the continual bombardment of physical stimuli. As a result, you'll be able to absorb this type of physical punishment with fewer injuries and quicker recuperation.

" "   TIKI BARBER

TRAINING WITH A PRO

I first met Joe Carini as I began my eighth NFL season with the New York Giants. By then I was comfortable with my role on the team, but less comfortable with my own personal development. Although I didn't think about it all the time, I knew I had to make some changes physically that would improve my performance. I needed a trainer who could help ignite my muscle development and turn me into a more powerful, explosive, and durable running back.

At that time my two best qualities on the field as a running back were my elusiveness and versatility. My opponents found it hard to catch me and hard to outguess me. But because I was always looking for extra balance, I'd use my arms—while holding the ball—to my body's advantage. This meant I could stay on my feet while sprinting, running, and twisting. But using your arm to break tackles or keep your balance means you have one less arm protecting the football, which is why I fumbled so much. I also knew I wasn't durable enough, so I avoided collisions with other players and sacrificed some of my effectiveness in the process. Knowing my weakness motivated me to change.

What I needed most was someone who could push me to find my potential, to remind me that strength and mental toughness had no limits. Joe Carini unleashed a side of me that I knew existed but didn't know how to access. He did this by unlocking the tenacity he knew I had, that drive that made me want to succeed. He propelled me past my preconceived limits.

Joe didn't just improve my strength; he changed my entire game. After an off-season of working out with him, I became explosive and powerful. I could run through tackles and deliver—and take—hits. My muscles were no longer lean, but layered, like a tightly wound rope. My joints, ligaments, and connective tissues became stronger and more durable. I was no longer afraid of getting hit. After working out with Joe, I became the complete player that I'd envisioned.

Joe and I developed the perfect partnership. If I ever had doubts about myself or my game, he was there to set me straight—with both weights and words. He was always calm and confident about his program, and in my body's ability to change. He helped me develop a real working relationship with my body that went beyond anything I had ever experienced before, even in the NFL. He quickly became one of my closest and most trusted friends. If I needed someone to jump in front of a train for me, Joe would do it (and he'd probably stop the train; he's that strong!).

Ultimately, Joe helped me improve my game by teaching me that failure just wasn't an option. He told me to delete the word "can't" from my vocabulary. Which is not to say I didn't fail at some lifts—I did—but I never questioned my ability to eventually succeed. It was all a process. And this mental toughness carried over to the football field. For the rest of my career, I never faced an opponent I couldn't best.

" " **JOE CARINI**

MAKING AN UNBREAKABLE ATHLETE

I first met Tiki Barber after he'd been an active player in the NFL for seven seasons. Tiki wanted to get strong, and he had the confidence and ambition to make that happen. He knew he could do better, but he needed someone to point out how to get there. During the four years prior to his beginning training with me, he fumbled thirty-five times. That wasn't acceptable to him, so we set about changing how he worked his muscles and thought about himself as an athlete. After he began working with me, and until he retired three years later, he fumbled only eight times. He put on about 20 pounds of muscle and for the final three years of his career showed the world that he was among the best running backs of his generation. At his peak, you could make the argument there was no one better at rushing and receiving than Tiki Barber.

I met Tiki through his manager, Mark Lepselter, who was looking for someone who could help Tiki improve his game by bulking him up, which would hopefully reduce his fumbling problem. Mark checked out my credentials by working out with me first to see how effective my workouts were and whether they exceeded more traditional programs. After he was convinced my workouts were the real deal, he brought Tiki to the gym.

On that first day, Tiki weighed 183 pounds. He had a small, light frame that I classified as a "hard gainer," meaning it was difficult for him to add muscle to his frame. The only strength training in Tiki's background occurred while he attended the University of Virginia with his brother, all-pro cornerback Ronde Barber. This was thanks to the great strength coach John Gamble, who was a world powerlifting champion and knew his training. The emphasis, however, was on the brothers' work in track and field.

Truth was, Tiki had almost no natural strength. During the first session, he leg-pressed 400 pounds for 3 reps, bench-pressed 240 pounds for a few reps, and squatted 315 pounds for a couple of reps. Granted, this is far more weight than the average person can lift, but for a professional running back it wasn't much. But compare these weights to a typical workout after three years of training with me: He increased his leg-press to 1,100 pounds for 3 reps, bench-pressed with assistance to 450 pounds, and safety squatted 785 pounds. Additionally, he deadlifted more than 500 pounds for 4 reps and got his weight up to 216 pounds of rock-hard muscle.

Tiki trained with me mostly during the off-season. He did get to lift at the stadium from time to time during the season, but his body was getting beat up in the day-to-day routine of practices and games. But once he started working out with me, the enormous strength he built during his months off carried him through the following season. For the most part, Tiki said he felt pretty good, even though he was getting 350 carries each year.

Tiki not only became much stronger, but he also became faster, which counters the belief that bulking up will slow you down. The combination of strength and speed gave Tiki the confidence and mind-set he needed to run through and around the power hitters on the field. Although he got banged around (he was, understandably, a frequent target when other players became aware of his new power),

YOU'RE IN GOOD HANDS

L est you think the authors of this book are all talk while you do the heavy lifting, the following stats will remind you that two record-breaking pros are setting you up with the most effective workout you'll ever come across.

Now that Tiki has made good on his promise to retire, we must all make do with the memories of some of his famous achievements. During his fantastic career as a Giants running back, he:

- Amassed 2,390 yards from scrimmage in a single season, the second most of all time.
- Was the third player to have 10,000 yards rushing and 5,000 yards receiving in a career.
- Was the first player with 1,800 yards rushing and 500 yards receiving in a season.
- Led the NFL in yards from scrimmage for two straight seasons.
- Finished tenth all-time in total yards from scrimmage for his career.
- Went out at the top of his game, setting records for most yards in a running back's final season (1,662) and most in a final game (234).

Speaking of heavyweights, Tiki's trainer Joe Carini shattered a few records himself. He was the first man in New Jersey to squat with an 800-pound load on his shoulders. His personal best is 905 pounds (that's within striking distance of half a ton), and around his New Jersey stomping grounds, he was the first man to bench-press 600 pounds. He was also:

- New Jersey's Strongest Man for six years running.
- New Jersey's powerlifting champion for three years.
- The first man in his state to powerlift 2,100 pounds combined.

Some of Joe's other bests include:

- A 470-pound Seated Military Press, an 810-pound Deadlift, a 670-pound Bench Press, and a 470-pound Seated Press.
- Power Clean at 340 pounds for multiple sets of 2 reps.
- Best Curl (while cheating or swinging) 310 pounds.
- Shrug 1,300 pounds for 3 reps, or 800 pounds for 30 reps.
- Squat on machine from bottom position 1,210 pounds for 2 reps.
- A Good Morning Exercise at 605 pounds for 3 reps.

SPECIALIZED ATTIRE AND LIFTING EQUIPMENT

Prior to 1990, only a couple of men in powerlifting history benched-pressed more than 600 pounds. These days, it's not uncommon for some lifters to bench-press more than 900 pounds, especially if they're wearing bench-press shirts. Today's competitive lifters often wear specialized clothing—such as canvas squat suits or denim bench-press shirts—which are permitted in some powerlifting sports. The rule of thumb is if you can bench-press 400 to 450 pounds raw (i.e., without a specialized shirt), then you can bench-press 700 pounds or better wearing the right bench-press shirt.

Joe Carini has never worn a squat suit or bench-press shirt, but he appears to be the exception to the rule. He's worn knee wraps and a belt, though, for heavy pulling movements. He believes it's up to the individual lifter to decide whether to wear specialized clothing. Novice lifters should concentrate on lifting without using any belts or wraps. This will to allow them to build their bodies at a realistic pace that won't risk injury.

he avoided serious injuries and never missed a game. The change in his attitude, not to mention his body, was noticeable to everyone.

Tiki was competitive and had the ambition to improve his game and condition. He was tough and mature enough to challenge himself to build up his body from head to toe through a vigorous, hard-core weight-training program.

I've trained many world-class athletes, and no one has ever had the iron will to succeed like Tiki. His abilities and willingness to work hard separated him from all the rest. He never made excuses, never complained, and never took a day off . . . just pure hard work to achieve his ultimate goal of becoming one of the greatest running backs in NFL history.

One of the things about Tiki I admired every day was his work ethic. When he was playing for the New York Giants, he'd be at the stadium by six thirty A.M. to practice, watch countless hours of football tape, and then come to my gym. I'd then drive him into the ground with our strength-training sessions. He always came back for that next heavy set, even more determined.

The more Tiki believed, the more force he generated during our workouts. I was always intense, always demanding. I asked Tiki to believe in himself and believe in me. A man of great character, he just had that inner drive that a lot of people don't have. During my many years of strength training and being in countless gyms, I've never seen anyone want to improve himself as much as Tiki. He gets it done, whether it's training, spending time with his family and friends, or working with one of his many charities. He's a committed individual.

In my opinion, what makes a great professional athlete is more than just talent. It takes self-confidence and willpower. It also takes a daily commitment to improve and excel. Tiki had all that, especially the willpower and commitment, but he had to learn to trust himself to gain self-confidence. Building his body and seeing it get stronger each week did just that. A pro athlete must impress the coach, competitors, fans, and spectators. Tiki understood that every word I said to him would improve his confidence—as would every set, rep, and exercise.

Tiki willingly accepted that the grueling workout program we developed would serve him on several levels. His body grew strong, strong enough to handle the punishment his sport dealt him. We never did any of the easy or soft workouts that some high schools, colleges, and even professional teams use. I'm all about real strength and bulk routines for gaining size and muscularity. And no shortcuts: People who pump steroids haven't a clue about the damage they do to their bodies and well-being. I don't think they have the courage to do it the right way—which is also the hard way. But Tiki did.

Tiki's story is an awesome one. Everyone talked about his amazing transformation; and because he's a star, it took on almost a magical significance. But the truth is, anyone can learn the proper way to train to get the same results. It's all explained in this book. If you're willing to put in the sweat equity, you can own a body as powerful and responsive as Tiki Barber's.

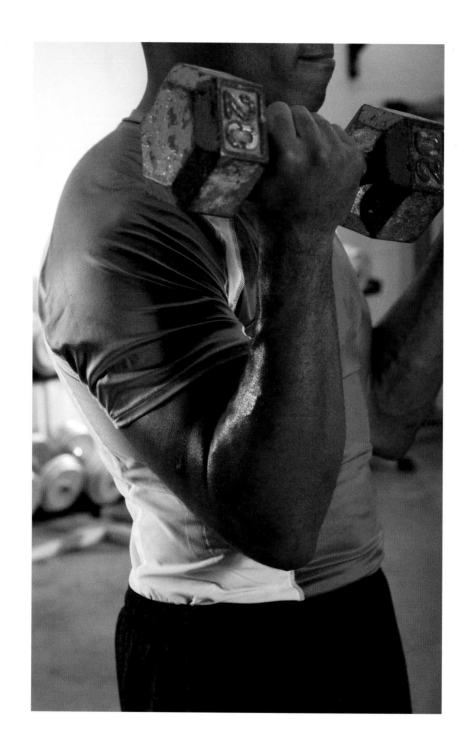

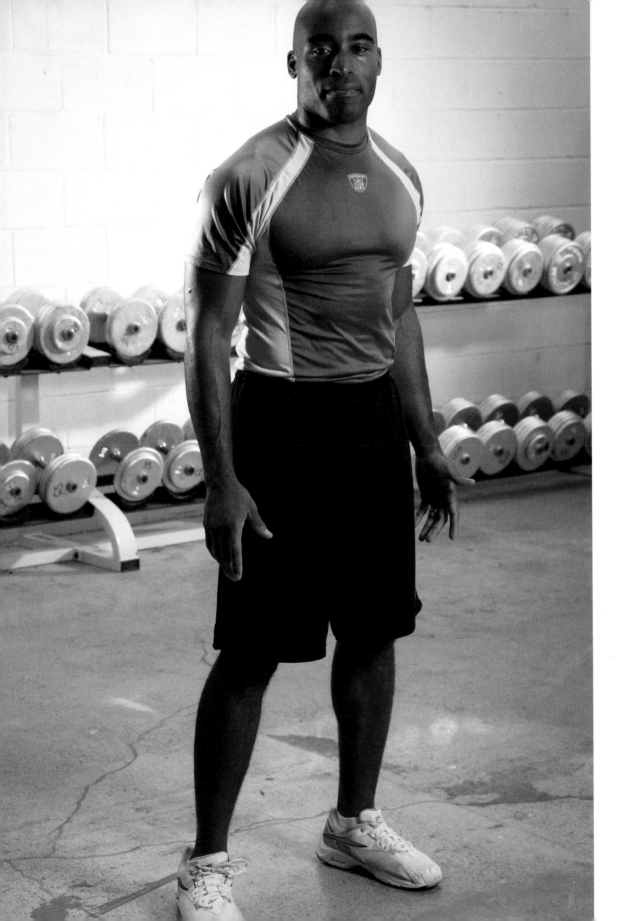

CHAPTER 2
THEORY AND EXECUTION OF POWERLIFTING

" " TIKI BARBER

The first step in my strengthening program involved moving from Nautilus equipment to free weights. My particular workouts—scrupulously true to the philosophy that if you're not lifting off the ground, you're not engaging brute strength—focused on core areas: legs, midsection, and upper body. I was never really a weight-room guy until I met Joe.

Sad to say, but most guys training today have no clue about how to build up their bodies—and before I met Joe, I was no exception. Believe it or not, we tend to be too soft about how we train. Modern weight-training programs pay almost no attention to making your tendons and ligaments stronger. Instead, they emphasize working the noticeable muscles in isolation. If your weight-training program focuses on muscles but ignores tendons and ligaments, it's still possible to get bigger and stronger. However, you won't even begin to reach the levels of strength you can achieve if you train your muscles, tendons, and ligaments as a unit. And while many programs will help you *look* strong, this one will give you functional strength.

And this leads to the subject of gyms in general. I think they're great places to get focused and do some serious body work, as long as you're aware of two things that often get in the way of that: machines and trainers.

You can't build tremendous strength on machines because they don't build up those stabilizers. The machines stabilize the weight for you, and thereby do half of the work. How often do you see people doing Deadlifts in commercial gyms? Not often, because many gyms don't even have weight-training rooms, and gym owners don't like patrons using chalk on their hands and spreading it around. They're not fond of grunting, either. And they're afraid that someone will get injured and they'll be liable. That's a shame because I've learned that a Deadlift is one of the best movements in weight training when it's done correctly. And for that, you need a really experienced trainer.

Many personal trainers these days are good at motivating their clients, but unfortunately, they probably have little or no knowledge of correct training procedures. With a training chart given to them by the gym, they walk around with their client for 45 minutes to an hour, marking off the exercises until the session is completed. After ten to twenty sessions of this, the client may not look or feel much better. That's because doing the same exercise with the same intensity just doesn't get the job done.

Take, for example, a man who's trying to gain weight. He'll do his 10 sets of biceps but skip the hard stuff—the leg and heavy back work. He can do 75-pound Barbell Curls but can't squat his own body weight for 20 reps. He and everyone else who trains like that lack the knowledge it takes to really bulk up. Compared to the legs and back, arm muscles are a relatively small percentage of your total muscle mass. It just makes sense to train your whole body so you add muscular weight everywhere. After all, that's the real goal. And I can tell you that it worked for me.

Power training is not bulk training. Many athletes believe that if they gain muscular body weight they will increase power. While this is true to a degree, it has no place in athletic competition, where it's more appropriate to gain strength without gaining added body weight. This allows you to increase your body efficiency, which ultimately should decrease added body weight. Unless you want to weigh 300 pounds or more, there's really no reason you should be adding large amounts of body weight.

To this end, when training for the three major power lifts—Squat, Bench Press, and

Deadlift—it's important to remember your end goal: big-time strength. There are many variations for each of those movements, which allow you to gain strength without going stale. With practice, you will develop the ability to recognize which exercises yield the best results.

All power lifts consist of pressing movements, squatting movements, and pulling movements. You need at least one of these three lifts in each of your workouts. What's important to remember here is that a powerlifting routine is not that complicated: Powerlifting consists of heavy, low-rep routines that allow you to gain the most muscle and the most power in the shortest amount of time. Yes, these exercises are physically demanding, which means you need to stay focused, stay confident, and work hard.

THE PHYSICAL ELITE OF SPORTS

To join the ranks of the physical elite of the sports world, you must train hard, heavily, and long. Most of us can't do this all at once, but that's what separates professional athletes from the weekend warriors. Most of us can train either hard or for long periods, but not both. It seems that the average person can't train heavily for long periods.

The brute-force workout described in this book will transform your life. You'll start by developing your ability to work out for long sessions. To adapt to a more intense workout, you'll start by learning to recuperate from repetition, building up from a few heavy reps. In time you'll be able to work out for long periods with at least medium-heavy resistance. No, there's no easy way out here. Somewhere along the line you must pay the price to earn the reward.

PROPER BREATHING

The most common mistake novice lifters make when starting out is not paying attention to their breathing. Most people don't know how to breathe properly when they're lifting.

For example, when many lifters lower the bar to their chests during a Bench Press, they don't breathe in and expand their chest cavities. This cuts off their air supply and limits their potential to increase the amount of weight they lift. In general, you should inhale during the lowering phase of a lift and exhale during the lifting itself. You might find that forcibly exhaling gives you a little extra "push" to move the weight.

You must learn to inhale and exhale through your mouth; this will allow your strength to work for you rather than against you while you lift. Holding your breath at any time during a workout isn't good for your overall health. When you breathe properly, your workout will be much more productive.

Obviously, your genetic makeup, personal lifestyle, and schedule will challenge this program. It will be a difficult road. You will have to believe wholeheartedly in yourself and your ability to revamp your mind-set and body. Tiki did it in three years, beginning when he was twenty-nine years old.

UPPER-BODY POWERLIFTS

The Bench Press is by far the most popular powerlift. It's been popular for years, even before powerlifting became an organized sport. Of all the heavy-lifting exercises, this one gives the most in terms of instant gratification. Bench Presses quickly build your upper body,

and they're not difficult to do. You lie down and push a barbell to arm's length above your chest. This will net you a big chest, and powerful shoulders and arms. After a few years of doing this exercise, you'll be able lift a substantial amount of weight, which looks impressive and feels pretty good, too. Faddish weight trainers are always asking each other how much they can "bench." They don't care how much you squat, deadlift, or military-press overhead. It's all about how much you can bench-press.

But the entire upper body—lats, chest, deltoids, triceps, and biceps—also must be developed fully and heavily. The *big* lifts—those that work the lats and chest—also help work the deltoids, triceps, and biceps.

THEORY AND EXECUTION OF POWERLIFTING

To motivate yourself for these difficult exercises, keep in mind that your back accounts for about two-thirds of your total chest measurement. Thus, if you want to increase your chest size, you should include exercises that build up your back. When your lower-back muscles are thick and strong, and your upper lats and trapezius muscles are well developed, you'll look and feel powerful.

CHEST

The best exercises for the pectorals are Barbell and Dumbbell Bench Presses from the incline bench, heavy Dumbbell Bench Presses, and Dumbbell Flys. By itself, however, the Bench Press will also develop the triceps.

UPPER BACK

The best exercises for the upper back are the Barbell Bent-Over Rows, Dumbbell Rows, Lat Pulldowns, Shrugs, Chin-ups, and Rows on the lat machine.

DELTOIDS

The exercises that work best for the deltoids are Seated or Standing Shoulder Presses, Presses behind the neck, and Push Presses off the rack.

TRICEPS AND BICEPS

The best exercises for the triceps are Standing Triceps Extensions, Triceps Lying Extensions, Lat Pushdowns, and Dips. Biceps can be developed through a vast range of barbell and dumbbell curling movements.

Beyond these core lists, "assistance movements" will aid in building your overall strength and muscular development. Assistance movements help to develop strength in other areas. For example, the Leg Press helps build a bigger Squat; the Close-Grip Bench Press for your triceps helps build up a bigger Bench Press for your chest muscles; Shrugs help build up your lower-back strength.

Assistance exercises help build your body *and* your lift. A great aid for the Bench Press is the Close-Grip Bench Press, which also helps build strong triceps and front deltoids. The more weight you can push during an assistance exercise, the more pounds you'll be able to lift during the main exercise. More poundage equals bigger muscles. Find an assistance exercise that works best for you, then add it to your program—but *not* as a replacement for the main lift.

Doing assistance exercises should never take the place of doing the actual powerlift. Always train your *big* lifts—Squats, Bench Presses, Deadlifts—then do your assistance movements. It's helpful to change your assistance work every few weeks to keep you from going stale. Just remember that we're not

SPOTTING

Gym courtesy suggests that you become a good spotter for other lifters. The golden rule applies: Spot for others as you'd like them to spot for you. This means keeping the lifter safe and giving your full attention while spotting. Here are some pointers.

Bench Press—The spotter or spotters should hand the bar off to the lifter, stand back, let the lifter perform his or her set number of reps, and then help replace the barbell in the rack.

Seated Dumbbell Press—The spotter should stand behind the person doing the Presses. Let him or her set in the number of reps, then grab the person behind the elbows and help with extra reps if needed.

Squat—It's helpful to use two spotters, who stand on each side of the squatter so if he or she fails, they can grab the bar to help the lifter avoid injury and return the weight to the rack.

talking the main lifts, here. Roughly 60 to 75 percent of your workout should come from assistance exercises with high repetitions (8 to 12) to build strength and endurance.

LOWER-BODY POWERLIFTS

Know first that the most powerful and largest muscle groups are in the legs. Once you've thoroughly strengthened those muscles, the power and bulk you'll achieve will last a lifetime. We can't overemphasize how important Squats and Deadlifts are to achieving overall strength and size. And here's something you might not know: Proper leg work and heavy squats will prompt your body to produce testosterone, which in turn helps you get bigger overall. Periodically during any workout, you should always squat or deadlift. Squats, correctly done, will build strength faster than the same reps of any other exercise.

Leg work is of the utmost importance and can determine whether you eventually reach your maximum potential. Hip and thigh movements, with most of the emphasis placed on various squatting routines, will transform your body beyond your wildest imagination. No matter what sport you're drawn to or if you just love to train, lower-body work will develop your physical condition to that of a champion athlete. Your legs can become so strong that almost any physical endeavor will be within your capability. In fact, such strength training will enable you to handle long, more intense workouts.

When training the lower body for greater physical conditioning, certain muscles should

TIKI'S
REGULAR-GUY WORKOUT

Want to get a feel for the massive poundage Tiki moved while in the NFL? Check out the sample workout week below. For detailed explanations of each exercise, see Part IV.

Day One: Just Get It Done
- *Leg Press:* 800–950 pounds, 2–3 reps
- *Squat:* 675 pounds, 3–10 reps
- *Good Morning:* 160 pounds, 7–10 reps
- *55-yard sprint:* while carrying a 300-pound weight, 7 reps
- *Hammer Bench Press:* 400 pounds for 1 rep
- *Incline Bench Press:* 380 pounds for 1 rep
- *Dip:* using a 90-pound belt, 7–10 dips
- *Arm Curl:* 55-pound dumbbell, 3 sets of 8 reps
- *Lying Dumbbell Kick:* 50-pound dumbbell, 10 reps

Day Two: Here's Something New
- *Hammer Press:* 360 pounds for 1 rep
- *Shrug:* 800-pound barbell, 7–10 reps
- *Floor Pull:* 295 pounds, 2 reps
- *Dumbbell:* work with 30 pounds, 10–15 reps
- *Triceps Extension:* 80-pound dumbbell, 3 sets of 8–10 reps
- *Weighted neck harness:* 25 pounds for 15 reps

Day Three: You're Almost Free
- *Floor Pull:* 405 pounds, 3 reps
- *Deadlift:* 500 pounds, 2 reps
- *Dumbbell One-Arm Row:* 120 pounds, 6–8 reps
- *Seated Dumbbell Hammer Curl:* 60-pound dumbbells, 6–8 reps
- *Flex work:* 10–12 reps

be emphasized to gain the most results in the shortest time possible. For instance, heavy leg work, two to three days per week, will revamp your metabolism to new heights of efficiency and ability. The overall results will include an increase in training drive as well as in your workload capability. Your ability to recuperate from heavy exercise will also be greatly enhanced.

Lower-body work stimulates the circulatory and metabolic systems, which enable you to develop greater muscle mass and definition, and muscle density. The blood is circulated to the working muscles at a faster rate, and this also has a carryover effect on the rate of muscular recuperation. The exercises that increase your circulation help you to develop the ability to pump the muscles with fewer sets and repetitions. This means the muscles will be operating at a higher level of efficiency, which in turn will help you develop greater gains in muscle size and athletic conditioning, given enough time, sweat, and determination.

The following list of examples should help you understand the process required.

SQUATTING MOVEMENTS

Full Squat: This exercise uses all the muscles of the lower extremities but especially the hips, lower back, thighs, and backs of knees.

Half Squat: This is a variation of the Full Squat in which you descend only halfway. It helps develop "lock-out power" for the full squatting movement and helps build confidence when using heavy weight.

Box Squat: In this variation you actually sit down on a bench, then stand back up. A favorite of many powerlifters, this exercise is essential as it makes use of the "rebound principal," which allows you to both explode and control the barbell, all at the same time. It also teaches you to rock forward and shift the hips under the bar.

Bottom Squat: You can do this exercise in a power rack. Set the bar at a full squat position. By starting from the bottom and fighting your way up, you develop a great initial drive when you squat. Helps develop tremendous hip strength.

All Other Squats: The Front Squat, Hack Squat, Sissy Squat, and Side Lunge Squat are not as valuable as the four Squat movements noted above for strength and power.

DEADLIFT MOVEMENTS

You can't hide a weak Deadlift. It's a lift of guts and determination, and affects every muscle group in the body. Like Squats, Deadlifts will increase overall muscle mass. This isn't by any means a quick-fix exercise. You must put in an enormous amount of work if you want to lift a respectable weight in this discipline. The payoff is that Deadlifts and their variations can give you overall body power and strength.

ASSISTANCE LOWER-BODY MOVEMENTS

A Leg Press, on the other hand, will simulate an Inverted Squat. You can build up great poundage, as well as greater muscle in the thighs, knees, ankles, and calves on the leg press.

The Hack Squat is a thigh builder and shaper; it gives your front thighs a good workout. Leg Extensions build muscle around your knees and front thighs. Leg Curls or hamstring exercises will build up the backs of your legs.

Too many trainees think that by doing just these three exercises they'll develop strength in their legs. Nothing could be further from the truth. These exercises are for shaping and moving blood into the legs, not for building tree-trunk thighs and calves. Some might say that it's better than nothing, but that's just an excuse to avoid doing some Squats and heavy Leg Presses.

Again, it's important to reiterate that no matter what type of sport you're working on, you'll never reach your full potential without hard, regular lower-body training. Intense, plentiful leg work will literally rewire your conception of what constitutes pure hard work. Stimulating your metabolism through vigorous leg training is key. Without this intense and worthwhile training, you'll have to settle for mediocrity. It's up to you to decide just what you want and where you wish to someday go.

For Tiki, heavy leg work and various assistance movements were both desirable and necessary. Developing explosiveness in his lifting training was important to his quest for increased flexibility and unadulterated strength. Of foremost importance for Tiki was developing steady strength. Although it was necessary to develop speed and flexibility to maximize Tiki's capability, strength was the number one reason for his tremendous success. It can be yours as well.

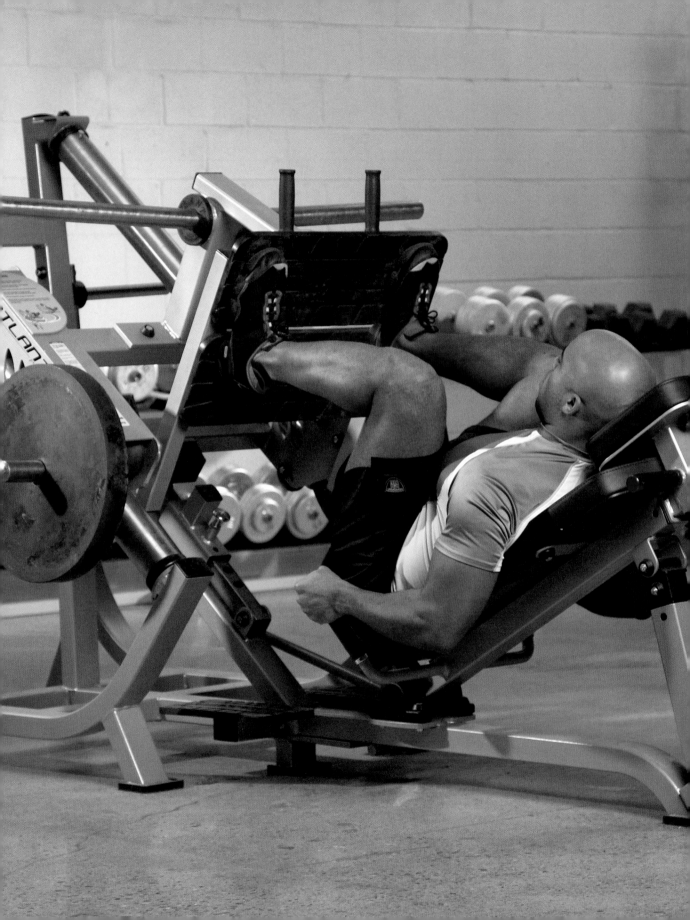

CARINI'S HOUSE OF IRON: LEAVE YOUR WHINING AT THE DOOR

News of a good thing always travels fast, and the word of mouth about Carini's House of Iron (carinishouseofiron.com) is that you'll walk out not only stronger but also equipped for success. Located in Pine Brook, New Jersey, the 12,500-square-foot gym has an unassuming look from the outside. Inside, however, is a carefully selected range of equipment that will increase clients' strength, speed, stamina, and flexibility.

But the gym's most important element is its sole proprietor and employee, Joe Carini himself. He's the inspirational dynamo behind all the success stories. Although House of Iron has been open only about a year—since October 2007—it already serves five hundred hard-working clients. People come here to train with Joe, and he makes sure that everyone leaves in better shape than they arrived.

Here's what he has to say about his power palace.

What's the significance of the gym's name?

Besides referring to weightlifting, the "iron" in House of Iron signifies a hard, impenetrable substance to emphasize the hard-core and very intense workouts that my clients do here. House of Iron denotes a gym where you train for strength and see how far I can push your limits. My gym and training methods aren't for the fainthearted. I want the name to challenge and remind my clients every time they walk through the door.

As a gym owner, what's your philosophy about training?

Train as hard as possible using the heaviest weights as possible. My goal is to coach each of my clients to achieve their personal best in fitness, no matter what their age, size, or condition. As the sole proprietor and employee, this means long workdays for me. I wouldn't be able to keep up the pace if I didn't really love what I do. I've been going strong for more than thirty years. Training and coaching others is all I've ever wanted to do, and I think that single-minded focus inspires my clients to reach beyond their limits and achieve goals they didn't think they could reach. The reward for me is seeing my clients claim their peak strength. Most of them apply their experience to other parts of their lives, knowing they can achieve more.

What sort of layout and equipment does the gym have?

The gym has everything necessary for balls-to-the-walls training. All the equipment is heavy-duty and built to last, whether it's a treadmill or strongman gear. In addition to the cardio machines, there are all kinds of strength-training equipment; safety squat bars, bands, and chains; power racks; steel logs and yolks for the farmer's walk; tires; kettle bells; and heavy dumbbells up to 200 pounds. The gym is equipped with a full-size boxing ring with heavy bags and a full-size octagon cage for martial arts. I've also installed areas for rope climbing and sled dragging. I cater to anyone looking for more serious training and less pampering.

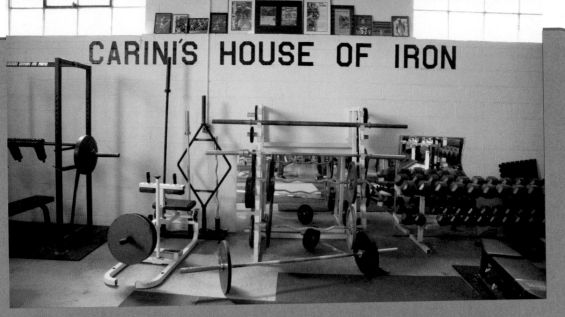

CARINI'S HOUSE OF IRON

Who else among the pro athletes uses the gym?

Besides Tiki, some of the pro athletes I've trained are Super Bowl champion and New York Giants center Shaun O'Hara, New York Giants guard Chris Snee, Carolina Panther defensive tackle Gary Gibson, Tampa Bay Buccaneer Luke Petitgout, Denver Bronco Paul Carrington, and others. In addition, many up-and-coming high school and college players train with me.

What are the first impressions of new clients walking into the gym for the first time?

They know immediately that they're in for some hard-core and serious training. People with athletic experience come to me knowing that I'll push them beyond what they've already done. New trainees are sometimes intimidated at first but soon realize that we're all there to reach our goals, so everyone fits in quickly. The atmosphere is serious but not elitist. If you're there to improve yourself, you're accepted. The pros are excellent role models and willing to help out the college and high school kids because they remember their own years as beginners. They know what it takes to elevate their games, and they're living proof that it can be done.

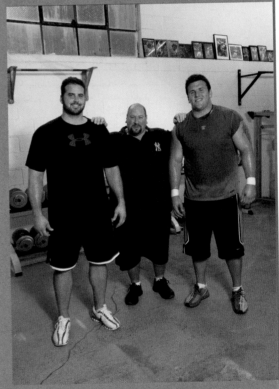

Joe and some of Tiki's former teammates and current clients of Joe: Shaun O'Hara and Chris Snee

Yes, you will need to warm up and stretch before moving into the powerlifting part of the program. A "cold" human body, like unheated plastic, can "crack" during movement if not warmed to sufficient pliability. Warm muscles loosen up better and stretch more easily. They also recover more quickly and are a lot less prone to strain or injury. Too, a full-body warm-up reduces the likelihood of one

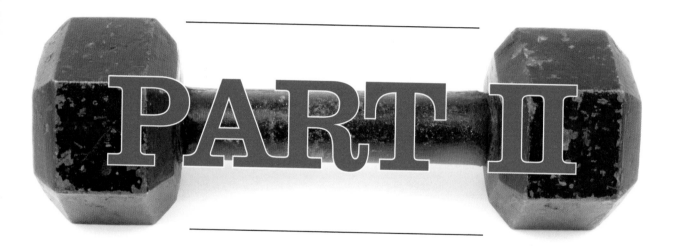

PART II

muscle remaining tight and causing a related muscle to strain in compensation.

The warm-ups described in this chapter also include stretching. Nothing too fancy, the exercises aren't intended for a contortionist but rather for the basic fitness buff, the man who's planning to engage in powerlifting and cardio conditioning several times a week, or even the man whose newfound commitment to pure hard work begins right here, with the stretching. —TIKI

GETTING READY FOR A PURE HARD WORKOUT

CHAPTER 3
WARM-UPS AND STRETCHES

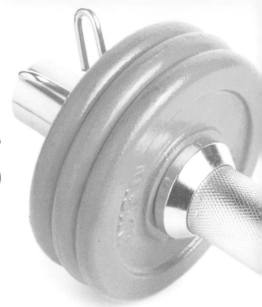

I n case you haven't heard, warm-ups aren't just for ballet dancers. Warming up focuses on two goals: gradually increasing your heart rate, and stretching your muscles to prevent injury. Walking briskly on a treadmill, riding a stationary bike, or jumping rope for five or ten minutes will take care of the first concern. Stretching your whole body, with emphasis on those muscles that you intend to concentrate on during the workout, will take care of the second.

Doing both before a workout is a good warm-up for anyone.

When you warm up, you prepare your muscle and connective tissue to be more pliable, to respond to the heavy-duty lifting portion of a workout without strains and pulled muscles. Your heart and lungs step up their pace, pumping blood and oxygen throughout your system. The capillaries feeding the working muscles dilate to bring more oxygen and fuel and remove more waste products. Sweating engages the body's cooling mechanism to prevent overheating.

A properly warmed-up body is one that's ready to train hard. You'll be able to focus more on the task at hand, and little pains and minor injuries aren't likely to hold you back from accomplishing your workout. Warm-ups and stretching get you set up for the coming workout and get your mind in the right place for the entire training session.

The danger of not warming up properly is injuries. It's never a good idea to try lifting maximum or near-maximum weights without warming up first with lighter weights. Attempt a big lift with a cold body and you're going to get hurt, which will result in missed workouts and more time before you can try that weight again.

Always warm up the specific muscles you want to train that particular day. A warm-up is also a good time to include practice reps of new movements, which you'll want to do slowly, concentrating on doing them perfectly. This is an excellent way for your body to learn new movements and adjust to them.

FLEXIBILITY

Stretching is important before and during exercising. The goal of stretching is to elongate and relax the muscle, and let the blood flow. Each person must discover which muscles need the most work. Lower-back muscles tend to tighten up for just about everybody, but the stretching focus for a basketball player, for example, will be different from the stretches a football player needs. Once you discover your body's particular requirements, it will be easy to work out your own routine of stretches.

Greater flexibility generally means greater strength because the muscles and joints are less restricted by stiffness and will work with increased efficiency. Full range of movements allows full contraction of the muscles, thus aiding in their development.

Flexibility is also essential to joint movement because it can help the joint generate maximum force. To truly develop your utmost potential in your lifting, you must have muscle flexibility. Tight, stiff muscles will lead to incorrect lifting styles and contribute to bad technique. Ultimately, this decreases your ability to lift a weight.

The importance of flexibility is that it allows a person to move without restriction. The real definition of flexibility is the ability to move a joint through a range of motion. Full range of motion can be influenced by many factors, including the type of exercise and connective tissues around a joint. Sometimes full range of motion is thought of as moving a joint beyond its safe range to stress a muscle or muscle group. But the stress in this case is applied to a muscle and has less to do with range of motion.

In addition, the tightening of any muscle groups will eventually lead to a decrease of muscle explosiveness, as well as a decrease of nerve fiber stimulation. A short, tight muscle won't bend when the extreme extension of lifting lasts for too long a period of time. Instead, it will snap. A tight, inflexible muscle means that the lactic acid won't be filtered out as quickly as possible after a hard workout, and this will mean muscle pain.

But don't get too crazy with your warm-up. Some people try to do too much stretching and actually hurt themselves. You must ease into a good stretching program. Overstretching, like lifting weights that are too heavy, can cause serious damage. So ease into a few minutes of stretching before a workout and wind down with several more minutes after your routine.

Make sure your flexibility routine isn't so intense that you become fatigued before your actual workout. As a general rule, the more intense the workout, the longer it will take to get loose. You should design a flexibility routine based on the muscle groups you intend to train—as a general rule 1 to 2 sets per exercise. Make sure the loads and reps used on any resistance movement are light enough to avoid fatigue.

After completing this routine, all your joints should be lubricated and ready to work out. You should perform 1 or more sets for each exercise. For lower-intensity workouts, you may need only a single warm-up set. Heavier workouts may take more.

Before you begin a training session, you should start with 10 minutes of cardio to get your blood flowing and your muscles loosened. Follow this with 5 minutes of general stretching,

choosing exercises for those body parts you'll be working that day. For example, if you'll be working your legs, do leg and back stretches to get warmed up. Instead of doing the same stretches repeatedly, choose several of them that are appropriate for each muscle group.

A SIMPLE WARM-UP ROUTINE

Neck Roll: Slowly move your head left and right, forward and back.

Arm Swing: Cross arms in front of your chest and then swing them down to your sides.

Wrist and Ankle Rotation: Make slow circles, clockwise and counterclockwise, to limber up the joints.

Rotator Cuff Swing: Shrug your shoulders up and down, then hold arms out to your sides and swing them up and down, and forward to back.

Toe Touch: Bend from the waist and touch your toes with your fingers. If you can't reach, stretch as far as you can without creating searing pain in your hamstrings.

Side Bend: Lean first to the left, then to the right, keeping your torso from bending forward or back. You can place your hands on your hips, or on the side that you're stretching, then raise that arm over your head as you perform the stretch.

Overhead Reach: Reach as high as you can above your head with your right hand, extending your arm as if you're trying to pick an apple off a high branch. Repeat with your left hand.

Trunk Twist: Clasp your hands at chest level, elbows bent, and twist your torso slowly and smoothly to the right. Then twist similarly to the left. You can increase the pace once your muscles have warmed up.

Hip Rotation: Circle your hips as if you're working a hula hoop, only keep the pace smooth and moderate. Change directions and rotate the other way.

Chin-up Bar Hang: Keep your arms fully extended.

Knee Lift: March in place, alternating raising each knee as high as it will go. You can increase the pace once you've warmed up to it.

A FULL-BODY WARM-UP ROUTINE

Jumping Jack: A quick and effective way to get the blood flowing throughout your body.

Body-Weight Squat: Do these without weights, concentrating on perfect form.

Push-up: Hold yourself above the floor with your arms straight, palms flat on the floor and shoulder-width apart (or wider). Hold your feet together or slightly spread apart. Inhale and bend your elbows to bring your torso near the floor. Avoid extreme hyperextension of your spine. Push yourself back to an arms-extended position, exhaling as you complete the movement.

Lat Pulldown: Sit facing the machine and wedge your knees under the restraint pad. Take a wide, overhand grip on the bar. Inhale and pull the bar down to your upper chest, arching your back and bringing your elbows back. Exhale as you complete the movement. Use light weight—remember, you're just warming up.

Sit-up: Lie on your back with your legs bent and your feet on the floor. Place your hands behind your head. Inhale and curl your torso off the floor. Exhale as you complete the movement. Return to the starting position without resting your torso on the floor.

Back Extension: Lie facedown in the Roman chair with the ankle supports properly adjusted and your hips on the support pads. Start with your thighs flexed and raise your upper body to a position parallel to the floor. Be sure to keep the proper arched position to reduce the chance of injury to the lower back. Excellent for stretching all the back and buttocks muscles.

COOL DOWN

The cool-down phase of the workout has a different goal from the warm-up. It's designed to bring your heart rate back down to normal. It's also a sort of decompression time to change your mental focus from training back to your everyday life. This is a good time to do some static stretching if you need to work on your flexibility.

Research has shown that static stretching—that is, moving a joint to a specific point and holding the position for a specific time—before any activity that requires a high-force output may actually make you weaker. Saving it until the end avoids this problem, and static stretching at this time typically allows you to stretch farther because your muscles are warm.

A cool-down routine doesn't have to be long. Five to 10 minutes is all that's required, depending on how much stretching you do. Start with a few minutes of walking, concentrating on your breathing. Keep track of your pulse. When your breathing and heart rate come down most of the way, stop and do some basic joint swings and rotations. Finish with a full-body static stretch. You should perform static stretches slowly and without bouncing. Go to the point of discomfort, not pain, and hold that for 15 to 25 seconds. Do 2 or more sets if you really need to work on your flexibility.

STRETCHES

Shoulder Stretch: Pull each arm across your chest and hold it with the other arm.

Triceps Stretch: Raise your bent arm up beside your head and pull your elbow back with the other arm.

Pectoral Stretch: Stand in a doorway and grab both sides with both hands, or grab a stationary object with one hand, lean forward, and let the weight of your body stretch your chest.

Side Bend Stretch: In a standing position, put one arm over your head and lean to the side, keeping your chest up.

Calf Stretch: Stand with one leg forward facing a wall. Keep your back leg straight and your back foot flat on the floor while you press on the wall and bend your front knee.

Seated Split Stretch: Sit with your legs open wide; stretch by reaching first over the left leg, then over the right leg.

Spinal Twist Stretch: Sit with one leg straight and the other bent. Cross your bent leg over your straight leg, put your opposite elbow on the outside of the bent leg at the knee, and attempt to turn and look behind you.

Piriformis Stretch: Lie back with both legs bent. Cross the right leg over the left so that the right ankle rests on the left knee. Grab behind your left hamstring with both hands and pull the knee toward your head. Repeat with the other leg.

Hurdler Stretch: Sit with one leg straight and the other tucked in. Lean forward and grab your straight leg or foot.

Quadriceps Stretch: Lie on your side, bend your top leg back at the knee, grab your foot, and pull your knee backward.

Cobra Stretch: Lie flat on your stomach, put your hands on the floor, and push your upper body off the floor; arch your back and look forward or up.

CHAPTER 4
CARDIO FOR A STRONG HEART

" "   **TIKI BARBER**

Lifting requires a strong heart, and the best way to keep this critical muscle a happy contributor to the program is through cardiovascular activity. When someone engages in any sort of exercise—be it lawn mowing or breaking tackles—stress is placed on the muscles as they're roused from their slumber and forced to actually *work*. This requires oxygen, lots of it, and at such times it's the heart's job to pump harder and faster, driving additional air through the lungs,

sending oxygen into the bloodstream and out to the protesting muscles. So long as the exercise continues, these working muscles will demand more oxygen, requiring the heart to regularly and rhythmically pump at an elevated rate.

Cardio also helps with recuperation and flexibility. Take a Strongman competitor or rock climber as an example. If neither had the cardio conditioning required for his sport, he wouldn't be too successful. Both would be prone to injuries, and they'd be stiff most of the time. Cardio exercising doesn't mean a person ends up gasping for air, but it does mean getting in good physical condition.

BEGINNER CARDIO EXERCISES

When a beginner starts cardio work, consideration must be given to overall physical condition. If you're overweight, start with 25 to 45 minutes of continuous low- to moderate-intensity work at 60–70 percent of your maximum heart rate on your choice of cardio machine, treadmill, or stationary bike. It's important not to cut yourself short, though. Cardio workouts can be boring, and unless you're under medical orders that advise otherwise, it's important to provide variations to your routine. You need to be imaginative with cardio work. Mix in some boxing, martial arts, or Strongman events.

If you do 30 minutes on a stair climber at a moderate pace, you'll get sweaty and out of breath. This may do absolutely nothing, though, for your performance in a certain sport; these require different muscle groups and energy expenditure. To train a particular group, you must choose specific conditioning methods.

For beginners, your choice of exercises will depend on available equipment and training goals. Any exercise that gets your heart and breathing rate up will promote cardiovascular development. But muscles that aren't used in the training activity will receive little benefit. If your goal is sport-specific conditioning, you should emphasize movements and exercises most like those you execute in competition. If you're not training for a specific sport but rather for all-around conditioning or fat reduction, include a wide variety of exercises.

Running, swimming, rowing, cycling, calisthenics, hitting a heavy bag, and weightlifting are all suitable exercises for beginners. Anyone just starting an exercise program should keep a training journal. Successful training is the result of a multitude of factors. A training journal can help you track your progress, and identify strengths and weaknesses. It will also keep you focused on your goal. Include detailed information about each of your conditioning sessions. Document how your mind and body are responding to each movement. Go over everything in your mind. Ask yourself if the exercises and workout are bringing you closer to your goals, your diet and supplementation schedules, and your progress.

You should make time for a brisk 20 to 25 minutes of cardio exercise three to five days a week, especially if you're also doing heavy lifting. You can do your cardio either on days you lift or on your days off; it's up to you. If you can get to the gym only three days a week, then you'll probably have to do some of your cardio on the days you lift weights.

PUMP AT AN ELEVATED RATE

Most everyone believes that walking or using a treadmill, bicycle, or elliptical machine is good; some would even say it's excellent. But nothing compares to cardio using extra resistance. When people use just their own body weight during cardio exercise, their bodies eventually adapt to the stress involved, and they begin to get decreasing benefit from it. Even if you're adhering to a strict diet, your metabolism and body chemistry won't get the most benefit from a cardio workout unless you include additional resistance in the mix, for example, walking with a weighted vest. Whether you're a man or a woman, if you get bored with the conventional cardio exercises, try the following variations:

Treadmill: Run or walk for 20 to 40 minutes with a weighted vest, ankle weights, or dumbbells.

Bicycling: Try 20 to 30 minutes with a weighted vest.

Medicine ball: Throw it around for 20 minutes. Or walk or run to it, pick it up, and repeat the maneuver for 15 to 20 minutes.

Barbells on the shoulders: Walking with heavy weight is an excellent exercise for anyone who's interested in strength development. Most human movement takes place in a standing position, so it makes sense to work all the muscles in the body from this position.

INTERMEDIATE AND ADVANCED CARDIO EXERCISES

Intermediate and advanced athletes typically prefer a more objective measure of exercise intensity, and that's their heart rate. There's a direct relationship between how hard you work and how high your heart rate goes.

Working muscles need heavy blood flow to bring oxygen and fuel and remove metabolic waste products. Your heart meets this demand by pumping harder and faster. When you first begin exercising, even mildly, there will be a rapid jump in your heart rate. If you continue working at that pace, your heart rate will quickly level off and possibly even drop slightly into what is called a steady state. At this point, slight increases in intensity yield slight increases in heart rate. Therefore, different percentages of your maximum heart rate will correspond to different percentages of maximum intensity.

How do you determine your maximum heart rate? The following equation provides a reasonably good estimate:

Maximum heart rate = 220 – Your age in years

Once you've figured out your maximum heart rate, your workout intensities can be quantified as percentages. For example, if your maximum heart rate is 190 beats per minute (bpm), then 60 percent of that rate would be 114 bpm, and you'd want to monitor your working heart rate to make sure you stay within that limit.

There are three different methods for determining your working heart rate:

1. Heart rate monitor: A monitor has a chest strap that you wear under your shirt. It detects your pulse and transmits it wirelessly to a watch. Usually it measures and transmits every 10 seconds or so.

2. Heart rate device: This measurement device looks like a stick with metal handles and a display in the center. You grab the handles, holding the device for 10 to 15 seconds, and it displays your heart rate measurement. Most modern cardio machines have heart rate devices built in.

3. Low-tech counting method: Find your pulse in your wrist using your first and second fingers (your thumb has a pulse of its own and can throw off your count). Press lightly into your wrist until you feel your pulse. Starting at zero, count the number of beats in 15 seconds. You will need a watch or clock with a second hand to keep track of the time. Once you have the beats in 15 seconds, multiply that number by four to calculate beats per minute.

It usually isn't possible to check your pulse during hard exercise. If you're wearing a heart rate monitor, you may be able to look down occasionally. If you have an expensive model, you can set the watch to beep when you go above or below a certain heart rate. Check your heart rate immediately after the work interval because it will drop quickly if you're in good shape. Here are some zones to consider:

Warm-up zone: 50–60 percent max heart rate (HR)
Low zone: 60–80 percent max HR
Medium zone: 80–90 percent max HR
High zone: 90–100 percent max HR

ADVANCED CARDIO: STRONGMAN WORKOUTS

What we call "strongman cardio" involves a series of hybrid exercises that increase your heart rate while working your muscles. There's nothing like them for burning calories and producing a big sweat. After one of these sessions, you'll feel like a million bucks. After a few months of them, you'll look like a million bucks, too.

Strongman cardio exercises include pulling a sled, pushing a car (yes, really), and carrying heavy objects for a certain time or distance. These exercises will get anyone in great cardio condition as they work the entire body from head to toes. Tiki actually did very little traditional cardio training in the off-season—no long runs or hours on the stationary bike. His strongman lifting with Joe was enough on its own to keep him in NFL shape. Strongman cardio is much more demanding on the cardiovascular system than walking on a treadmill, stepping on an elliptical machine, or riding a stationary bike.

Strength endurance training is so powerful a tool that these exercises will toughen not only your body but also your mind. When

AEROBIC VS. ANAEROBIC ENDURANCE TRAINING

Aerobic endurance is the ability to perform repetitive motions for a period of time greater than 3 minutes. Slow-twitch muscle fibers, which produce energy by converting fats aerobically, are adept at performing this type of contraction and use a specific energy system. Long-distance running, cycling, and soccer are just a few activities that incorporate large amounts of energy from the aerobic energy system and slow-twitch muscle fibers. These activities do use fast-twitch muscle fibers but only for brief outputs of strength.

If you're looking to build strength and size, however, long and slow cardio won't do much more than waste time. That's because this type of aerobic activity burns up too much testosterone, and that's counterproductive to developing size and strength.

Tests have shown that athletes who do a brisk 20 to 22 minutes of cardio will improve their heart rates and overall stamina, but longer periods won't improve their strength or size. However, when they run or walk with, for example, a sled or weighted harness, they gain not only size but also overall strength. This type of cardio workout is much more challenging for trainees. The results are measurable and should help them keep up their enthusiasm—and inspire them to continue.

Speed or speed aerobic endurance benefits other components of performance, allowing the body to work at an efficient level over a prolonged period of time. This training doesn't have to be daily but rather can be done three times per week at a lower target heart rate (say, 75 percent) to maintain cardiovascular fitness and aerobic endurance. If your goal is strength, then a high volume of aerobic endurance training will decrease the effectiveness of any form of strength training. The benefit of aerobic endurance training is that it leads to total fitness.

Anaerobic endurance—such as a wrestling match, downhill skiing, or 2 minutes of Push-ups—is a component of fitness that will benefit anyone who has a goal of strength and speed. Anaerobic endurance will aid in high-intensity output for a short period of time.

This type of training uses primarily blood glucose as the source of energy. Lactic acid buildup also occurs during this training, but increased conditioning can prolong the period of time before lactic acid levels get so high that muscular contraction will cease to occur. This also happens when an exercise is done for fewer than 10 seconds at an all-out effort. Anaerobic endurance training lengthens the threshold point, thus improving athletic and training performance. It can also be beneficial for individuals whose work may involve 1 minute of high output and 30 seconds of recovery. Circuit training, super sets, and alternate sets are a few training methods that can help increase anaerobic endurance.

you're fighting for survival, as these exercises simulate, you're also fighting your mind with your will. You're pumping blood, strength, and endurance through your veins while sweating fear, doubt, and poisons out through your pores.

During a strongman cardio workout, every muscle group comes into play. You'll burn more calories because you're expending concentrated effort in a short amount of time.

For example, it takes a lot more energy to do a farmer's walk—carrying 100 pounds for a quarter mile—than to just walk the quarter mile. When you flip a tire for a prescribed distance, every muscle group in your body is affected. The tire flipper will burn more calories during the same time period than, say, a bike rider for the simple reason that it takes more effort. If you're ready for a full-on strongman cardio workout, see chapter 15.

CHAPTER 5
A POWER-LIFTER'S FOOD GROUPS

"TIKI BARBER

Heavy lifting burns a tremendous number of calories each session, and although it's necessary to stay fueled, it's more important to invite your brain to the table along with your appetite. Choosing the right food at the right time can keep muscles growing at a steady rate and help prevent plateaus and exhaustion. When lifting heavy weights, you need strong bones and tendons. To this end, you must fuel your body with protein, carbohydrates, and

the good fats, but you definitely don't want to overeat or consume empty calories.

Nutrition—or the lack of it—is the number one reason your training will succeed—or fail. Some athletes claim nutrition counts for

as much as 80 percent of their success. And that means supplying your body with the right nutrition for the type of training you do. If your body doesn't take in enough calories from protein, the good kinds of fats, and carbohydrates, you will not develop and grow at the rate you should. Joe was constantly reminding me to eat, eat, eat, and it's a big reason why I got stronger. As you start lifting, you're going to find your appetite increasing—so eat up.

BALANCING THE KEY INGREDIENTS

For someone participating in serious power-lifting or athletic training and looking to get bigger, adding more calories to the overall daily caloric intake is the first and most important step. You want to aim for somewhere between 35–40 calories per kilogram of body weight. (To get your body weight in kilograms, simply divide your weight in pounds by 2.2.) A 220-pound person (100 kg), for example, should consume about 3,500–4,000 calories each day. If that sounds like a lot, it is. Best practice is to divide this into five or six small meals throughout the day, paying special attention to the pre- and postworkout meals (more on these later). (By the way, we use kilograms because that's how nearly all the scientific literature reports it; if you're more comfortable using pounds, the formula is 16–18 calories per pound of body weight.)

Don't be afraid of calories. As long as you're following through on your workouts, your food intake will complement your efforts in the gym. Trying to gain muscle and weight through exercise alone, without eating enough food, is essentially like trying to build a house without lumber or cement. If you want to add 10 pounds of muscle to your body, where do you think it's going to come from if you don't take in more food?

Nutrients in food not only provide energy for your body; they also supply the raw materials for increasing muscle mass—and building just about everything else in between. For instance, the carbohydrates in the protein bar you eat before your workout are converted into glucose, the quick fuel your muscles draw on while expending energy. After your workout, your body takes the meat in your sandwich and breaks it down into amino acids, many of which head directly to the muscle group you worked on earlier.

People who don't pay attention to a daily nutrition routine can end up with a variety of ailments. You must think—and eat—smart. You must learn to listen to your body and figure out what suits it best. To put on healthy body weight, you must consume wholesome foods, lots of protein, good carbohydrates, and the fats found in nuts and olive oil. This doesn't mean overeating or consuming empty calories; it means eating five to seven times per day, every day. If you develop good nutritional habits and goals, the benefits will add up quickly, and the results will be noticeable quickly.

When it comes to your diet, you must make some important decisions, set goals, and work to achieve them. You've heard it before, but here it is again: Aside from straight poison, refined sugar is the most harmful product you can put in your body. This may be a bit of an exaggeration, but don't miss the point. Refined sugars deplete you of strength and cause all kinds of health problems.

That said, carbohydrates remain the most important component of an athlete's diet. In fact, during intense activity, your body gets about 90 percent of its energy from carbohydrates. Limiting carbohydrates has been shown repeatedly to impair athletic performance. However, all carbohydrates aren't created equal, as demonstrated by the glycemic index (see the sidebar on page 40).

Staying hydrated by drinking plenty of water provides your body with numerous benefits. Water is the biggest component of your body, accounting for between 50 and 60 percent of your total body weight. Water helps to support all your body's tissues, including your joints and muscles. In fact, even mild dehydration can have a serious effect on muscular performance. The consensus recommendation today for water intake stands at nine cups of water per day for women, and thirteen cups per day for men (that's about three-quarters of a gallon per day). During your workout, a good rule of thumb is to try to consume about a cup of water every ten minutes.

A WORD (OR TWO) ABOUT PROTEIN

Although the body is fueled by carbohydrates, both complex and simple, athletes should also pay attention to how much protein they consume. Without this powerful nutritional dynamo, all the carbohydrates in the world won't increase your muscle mass. Protein is the building block for muscles and probably the most famous of the three macronutrients. Protein is comprised of different amino acids, some of which are considered to be essential to the human body (meaning that the body doesn't produce them in sufficient amounts to meet metabolic demands). The protein from your diet is used in a variety of metabolic processes ranging from supporting your immunity, to building joints and tendons, and building muscle.

There's a lot of confusion and misinformation about the proper amount and timing of protein intake for training. If you consume too little protein, your body won't be able to build any lean mass because it won't have its most important materials. Consume too much protein, and you'll wind up pissing most of it away, literally.

So what's the right amount? If you're trying to increase your size, then you should consume between 1.2 and 1.6 grams of protein per kilogram of body weight, or between 0.54 and 0.72 grams per pound of body weight. In other words, a 220-pound (100-kg) person should consume 118–160 grams (4–6 ounces) of protein at each meal. Studies have demonstrated that strength trainers who consumed inadequate amounts of protein were hindered in their muscle development, whereas those who consumed enough protein enhanced their muscle development. However, it's pos-

THE GLYCEMIC INDEX

The glycemic index is a measure of how fast sugar from foods can raise your blood glucose (i.e., blood sugar) level. Foods scoring high on the index will raise a body's glucose levels faster than others. These high rollers include refined sugars, carrots, white bread, baked potatoes, and sports drinks (e.g., Gatorade). Foods low on the glycemic index include complex carbohydrates—whole grains such as oatmeal and brown rice—as well as leafy vegetables. Both complex and simple sugars have their roles in fueling athletes, provided you use their glycemic index properties to your advantage.

Complex carbohydrates take relatively longer to affect blood glucose levels compared to their high-glycemic counterparts. Therefore, consuming complex carbohydrates about 2 to 3 hours prior to your workout can help fuel your body as you make heavy demands on it. Furthermore, right before your workout (within 30 minutes), a light snack with high-glycemic carbohydrates can help give you a quick boost.

Immediately following your workout, another light meal with high-glycemic carbohydrates can help replenish your body's stores of sugar. Following that up with a good meal complete with complex carbohydrates is a good practice to help support your recovery. However, make sure that the high-glycemic foods you eat are wholesome, and not simply soda and refined sugar.

sible to reach a protein "ceiling," where very high intakes result in no additional benefit. That's why the estimate of 1.2 to 1.6 grams per kilogram of body weight is helpful to serious weightlifters.

How should you translate that into actual meat and potatoes? A good rule of thumb is that a single serving of protein accounts for roughly 7 grams of protein. A "serving" is a fairly loose definition, but normally it's a 1-ounce portion of meat, a single whole egg (or two egg whites), 2 tablespoons of peanut butter, or three slices of bacon.

How your body absorbs nutrients depends on the quantity that's consumed at a given meal. Protein is no exception to this axiom: The percentage of total intake that's absorbed decreases as the total amount you've eaten increases. Thus, most of a small amount of protein will be absorbed, whereas an oversized serving will be poorly absorbed. In fact, experiments have shown that muscles will grow with a preworkout protein intake in the single digits of grams. That's like a teaspoon of peanut butter. Most athletes take in adequate amounts of protein from diet, so less is more when it comes to protein powders and such supplements. Twenty to 30 grams of supplemental protein per drink, one to two times per day, is an adequate amount. Anything more than that is a waste, because it'll just get flushed from the body.

Dairy foods are also a great source of protein as well as calcium and vitamin D. A single serving of dairy—1 cup of milk; between ¾ and 1 cup of yogurt, depending on type; or 1 ounce of cheese—has about 8 grams of protein. Also, there's no difference in protein content between whole, 2 percent, and skim milk, but overall, skim milk is a better choice since it has a much lower fat content.

Timing your protein intake can also be an important aspect of your training. Ingesting a small protein meal before training, just as you do carbohydrates, helps to enhance your gains. If you provide your body with sufficient amino acids right before your workout, you ensure that your body has enough protein to begin repairing and building muscle as soon as it can.

Protein powders are probably one of the most commonly used supplements by athletes. It's always best to try to meet your needs first through whole foods rather than dietary supplements. That said, protein powders work well because they're quick and convenient (no cooking; just add milk or water), and because their nutritional analysis is printed right on their labels, they eliminate the guesswork of figuring out how much protein you're getting with a given serving. There's no shortage of protein flavors out there, most of which are similar. Overall, if you find something that doesn't break your budget and has about 20 to 30 grams of protein per serving, then you should be fine.

However, there's no getting around the cardinal rule of nutrition that "fresh is best." This means your body will work more efficiently with real food than with processed powders and supplements. This goes for protein, too. The best kind is certainly animal protein, as compared to vegetable sources. But should you decide to incorporate a protein supplement in your diet, there's no ideal form. As long as you maintain a grams-per-kilogram-of-body-weight ratio that's suitable for your body, you should absorb enough protein for your needs. Any differences that might exist between protein types and their absorption ratios probably aren't clinically significant.

THE POWER OF AMINO ACIDS

Protein has a variety of functions and roles in the body. It's made up of a long string of amino acids, each of which has a particular property that helps to determine the function of the protein in question. There are twenty different amino acids, and these can be separated into three different categories.

The first and most important are the essential amino acids. These can't be made in sufficient quantities by the body (if at all), and therefore must come from food. The second type are the nonessential amino acids, or those that can be derived from other molecules in the body. The third group is the conditionally essential amino acids, or those that are essential only during certain stages of life (typically for newborns and children).

GLUTAMINE AND CREATINE

iki was blessed with amazing genetics and an unparalleled work ethic, and never needed to use supplements. But for many people, they can be helpful. Glutamine, the most abundant amino acid in the body, can help with recovery. Glutamine is a major fuel source for many body cells. If glutamine isn't present in sufficient amounts in your diet, it's possible that other protein sources in the body (i.e., your muscles) may be tapped to meet this demand. Therefore, having adequate glutamine in the diet, whether from food or supplements, may help prevent muscle wasting and support muscle repair after training. When it's not in a powder, glutamine is found in nearly all foods that contain protein.

Creatine is another extremely popular supplement and can be beneficial to those participating in strength and power sports. Creatine is considered an amino acid, but unlike glutamine, it's not considered an "essential" one. Creatine helps create the metabolic pathway that provides energy during short, intense activity. It's found mostly in proteins such as meat and fish. By supporting this metabolic process with creatine, you'll help your body to work harder, and ultimately achieve greater results in developing strength.

Creatine is unique in that the dosing regimen can be somewhat tricky. When first starting on creatine, begin with a "loading phase," or a heaping tablespoon per day. After five days, you can begin the "maintenance phase," or 1 teaspoon per day. Creatine is safe to use, so long as you stick with the recommended dosages, and you drink enough water. Some people experience some minor cramps and pains when taking creatine, but again, this can be alleviated or prevented altogether if you're taking in enough water. One final note: If you have a preexisting kidney condition, you should consult with your doctor before taking creatine supplements.

Some types of creatine are better than others and it's important to research the different pills and powders. In some cases, creatine capsules are filled with vitamins or minerals and are not what they're advertised to be. Overall, it's probably best to stick with name brands rather than some of the generics.

Keep in mind that your body will reach a saturation point in terms of how much creatine it can absorb. According to some studies, when this point is reached, creatine's beneficial effects on athletic performance won't increase with increased use. Moreover, once this ceiling is reached, the amount in your system will decrease gradually over about a month before it returns to presupplement levels. Thus, some argue for periodic intake of creatine, building up to the saturation point, then allowing it to taper off to the baseline level. However, from the standpoint of athletic performance, there's no evidence indicating that constant use of creatine is any better or worse than periodic use.

You can walk into any health food store or vitamin shop and find a wide selection from which to choose. But the best choice is developing a sound nutritional program. Make it your goal to find out what diet best suits your needs, what you need from the food you eat. Supplement your diet carefully, reading all labels on the products you intend to use. Stick with a good multivitamin and mineral supplement. Incorporate some protein powder into your diet. If you're a strength athlete, find the right creatine and use it correctly.

Proteins can be classified into two basic groups: complete and incomplete. A complete protein is one that contains all of the essential amino acids in sufficient amounts, and an incomplete protein is one that doesn't. Complete proteins are derived mainly from animal sources, and incomplete proteins come from vegetables and grains (with soybeans a notable exception). By including multiple vegetable protein sources in the same meal, you can compensate for the amino acid deficiencies that occur in the individual sources. This practice is referred to as using "complementary proteins."

CHOLESTEROL, FATTY ACIDS, FIBER, AND SALT

Heredity also plays a critical part in your diet plan. If your family history includes certain illnesses such as diabetes and high cholesterol, you'll be at greater risk when you consume foods that encourage these conditions. Low-density lipoprotein (LDL) is known as "bad" cholesterol. High-density lipoprotein (HDL) is known as "good" cholesterol. You want to keep the HDL up, through proper nutrition and exercise, and the LDL down, to reduce the stress on your cardiovascular system and prevent heart disease.

Dietary approaches to maintaining a healthy cholesterol level include avoiding foods high in saturated and trans fats, while incorporating some of the good polyunsaturated fats into your diet. A simple way to identify saturated fats is by seeing whether they're solid at room temperature. Butter, lard, and vegetable shortening are all on the saturated fat list. Unsaturated fats are those that remain liquid at room temperature, typically oils such as olive oil, canola oil, and flaxseed oil.

Omega-3 fatty acids are believed to be responsible for the benefits associated with eating fish. These fatty acids primarily come from fish higher up on the food chain, such as salmon, tuna, trout, swordfish, and halibut. Omega-3s are great for your heart. In fact, the American Heart Association recommends eating fatty fish at least twice per week to help prevent heart disease.

In direct contrast to the damage that saturated fat can do, foods high in fiber can promote a healthy heart and lower your cholesterol. This is in addition to fiber's better-known role of regulating digestion. Foods high in fiber include whole grains, fruits (particularly dried fruits), and vegetables.

Blood pressure is normal or good at 120/80. Anything over 140/90 is considered high. To keep your blood pressure low, make sure you eat right, exercise, and avoid high-sodium foods. Too much sodium in a diet will contribute to high blood pressure. High-sodium foods include processed foods, canned soups, and some cold cuts (e.g., cured meats like ham and salami).

Throughout Part III, you will be introduced to all the various powerlifting exercises that helped shape me into a faster and more powerful running back. Some of these exercises may be familiar to you, while others were designed specifically by my trainer Joe Carini. Before the lifts you'll find a thorough

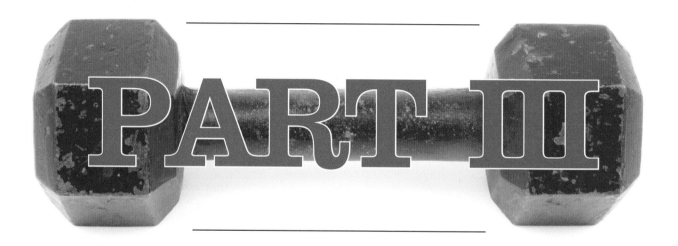

PART III

explanation of all the muscle groups and their functions, so you'll be able to picture the areas as you exercise. Knowing the anatomical differences between the muscle groups will keep you focused on the lifting technique, and also help you feel the difference as your muscles strengthen. Understanding your body and the ability to increase its level of performance are keys to a successful workout. →

DOWN
TO
PURE
HARD
WORK

In the beginning, you are training the mind as well as the body. The mind, after all, motivates you to train. The secret is to make your mind work for you. This means maintaining a positive outlook on your abilities and setting higher goals for your workouts.

Joe and I can't encourage you enough to read and understand the lifting technique of each exercise. Nothing impedes progress more than poor technique, especially when it comes to some of these powerlifting exercises. Even if you think you already know how to execute, say, a Leg Curl, you should try these movements slowly, with minimum weights, so you familiarize yourself with the techniques before adding the heavy-duty guys.

—TIKI

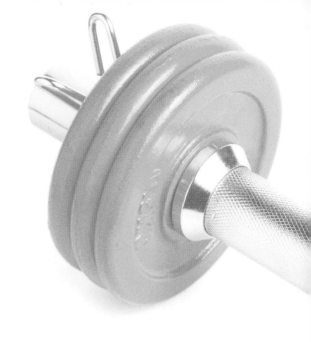

CHAPTER 6
THE MUSCLE GROUPS

There are hundreds of muscles in the human body, but for the purposes of lifting, you can think of them in five groups: Legs, Chest, Back, Shoulders, and Arms. Knowing a little bit about how these muscles work will help you make these muscles stronger.

LEGS

There are a total of thirty-seven muscles in your legs—twenty-two muscles work the hip joint, and fifteen work the knee joint. Your butt alone includes nine separate muscles. Some of these muscles draw the thighs apart; others flex the hip and rotate the thighs inward.

Don't worry too much about their names, but it will help your workout if you understand their separate functions.

The biggest muscle (the gluteus maximus) forms much of your butt. It's an important extensor of the hip, for it supports the torso in the erect position. You use it to rotate your thigh

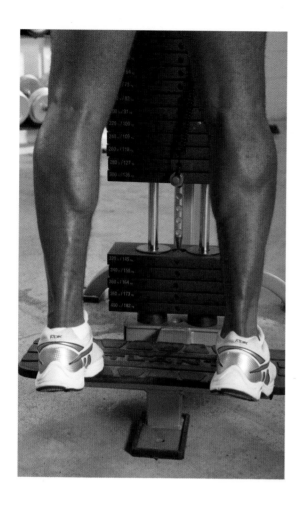

draw your thigh backward. When your knee is bent, they act to rotate your lower leg.

All these muscles work in various combinations so that you can bend or straighten your knees; move your thighs forward, backward, sideways, or toward each other; or rotate your thighs inward or outward. The hamstrings are particularly important to athletes because when you run, your forward movement in stride comes from the hamstrings, glutes, and calves.

Your calf muscles are the most difficult part of the body to develop. Health and fitness experts have advanced many theories for why this is, but most agree that no one specific factor can explain why some people have well-built calves and others don't. Genetics undoubtedly is the main reason, but then genetics is a broad term that includes, among other things, a person's natural tendency to develop the size and shape of his muscles.

We use our calves throughout the day, every day. From walking to lifting weights, we tend to take them for granted—at least until one of them gets injured. Then, as when you bang your thumb with a hammer, you're suddenly aware of how often you use these muscles, and just how critical they are for physical movement, especially in athletic pursuits.

outward. It acts mainly to draw the thighs apart, but it can also rotate your thigh inward.

On the front of your thighs is your quad muscle, which is actually four muscles that work together to help you straighten your lower leg and align it with your thigh.

At the back of your thigh are the three hamstring muscles. Your *hammies* flex the knee joint—that is, bring the lower leg back and up toward your thigh. The hamstrings can also help you extend your hip joint or

CHEST

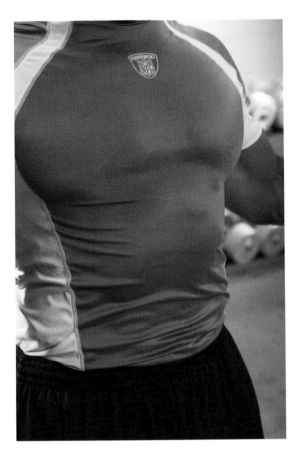

The framework of your chest muscles is similar to an open basket made of bone. At the back of the basket is the vertical column of your spine, where your ribs are attached. The bony chest is made into a closed box by two sheets of muscles, which facilitate the movement of the size and shape of the chest during breathing. As a result, the air is moved in and out of the chest.

The principal function of chest muscles is to draw your arms downward, inward, or forward. When your arms are fixed overhead, as when you're doing Chin-ups, you'll use your pectorals to draw your trunk upward. When you're benching, your pecs push the weight away from your body. Any muscle group that's used to make fundamental arm movements—such as movements brought about by the pectoral muscles—is of course critical in many sports.

BACK

Your back is almost entirely covered by a muscle called the latissimus dorsi, commonly called the lats. There are two sets of muscles that contribute in forming the back part of the armpits and govern the shape of the sides of the back. The main function of these two pairs of muscles is to draw the arms from overhead downward, and backward to the sides. The deep muscles of the back form a broad, thick column extending from the sacrum to the skull. Many muscles of varying length contribute to the mass. The largest of the deep back muscles extend or hyperextend the spine. In addition to the long muscles of the back there are a number of short muscles. These short muscles work together in extension and rotation of the spine and as spine stabilizers.

The spine muscles on a strong person's back will stand out like steel cables running from the butt to the neck. They extend and

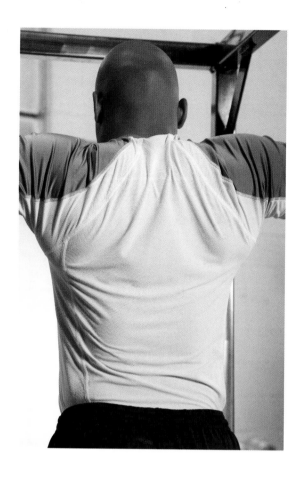

straighten the spinal column, and rotate the trunk. Lats also give you that V shape when viewed from the front and rear. They are big, powerful muscles when properly developed. Chin-ups, Pull-ups, Lat Pulldowns, Deadlifts, Bent-Over Rows, and Shrugs all build the lats.

SHOULDERS

The chief muscle that forms the cap of your shoulder is the deltoid muscle. When viewed from the side with your arm hanging down, the deltoid looks roughly like an inverted triangle

at the top of your arm. The base of this inverted triangle, which is the origin or top border of the deltoid muscle, consists of the outer third of your collarbone and the upper and outer borders of your shoulder blades and their apex. The deltoid points down and is formed by fibers converging into a thick tendon, which fastens to the bone of the upper arm about midway between the shoulder and elbow joints.

The deltoid's principal function is to raise your arm. The muscle consists of three portions: front, side, and rear. When the front portion acts, it raises the arm upward and forward. The side portion raises it upward and sideways, and the rear portion raises it upward and backward. The arm can be raised to the greatest height in front. When you move your arm directly backward, you usually can't raise it much beyond a forty-degree angle.

The deltoid's responsibility for raising your arm ends when your arm reaches the level of your shoulders or slightly above. From there on up, the raising is carried on by muscles that rotate your shoulder blade, carrying your arm with it.

One of the largest and most important muscles of the neck and shoulder region is the trapezius, which runs from the back of your lower skull down to the middle of the back and out to your deltoids. The traps assist in raising the arms (as in pressing a weight) from the level of the shoulders to overhead. Another function is to squeeze the shoulder blades together as when the shoulders are

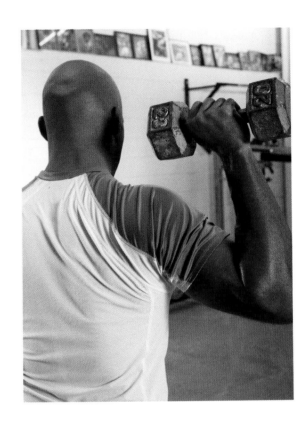

strength. Rotator cuff injuries, shoulder imbalance, and pinched nerves require the athlete to strengthen the shoulder area by rehabilitation, physical therapy, and reducing damaging activities. Exercising to ensure good shoulder strength will minimize injuries. Strong shoulders are also essential for holding heavy weights—whether you're pressing dumbbells or squatting with a bar. The shoulder area also assists when your hands are holding a heavy Deadlift.

drawn backward. The right and left halves of the trapezius unite in the middle of the back and form an extensive kite-shaped muscle.

Shoulder strength is of far greater utility and importance than upper-arm strength because your upper-arm muscles act on the elbow joint, whereas the deltoid muscles act to move your whole arm. For this reason, the deltoid bears to the arm the same relationship that the hip and buttock muscles bear to the thigh. In all overhead lifting—pushing forward, pulling backward, or forcing your arms sideways—your shoulder muscles are doing the work.

Football, baseball, weightlifting, boxing, wrestling, basketball, golf, and hockey are just a few sports that rely on shoulder

ARMS—TRICEPS, BICEPS, AND FOREARMS

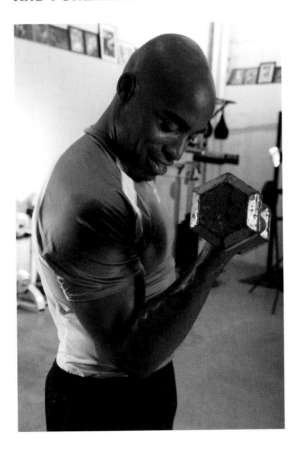

The triceps is composed of three muscles that make up the back of your upper arm. The triceps is an extensor of the elbow and thus performs a straightening function. This muscle group is responsible for all pushing movements with the arms. Strong triceps act as powerful forearm extensors. They're key to all pressing movements. In football, for example, strong triceps help a person throw a stiff-arm block or push off an offensive lineman.

The biceps—that swollen bulge on a fit person's arm—is one of the most recognizable muscles in the body. But it's actually two muscles that work together to bend the arm at the elbow. Anytime you pick something up or engage in a tug-of-war, your biceps comes into play.

When we think of big forearms, we often think of a person with hand strength and a strong grip. The forearm muscles close the hand or clench the fingers. Those muscles that open the hand, or straighten the fingers, are located on the thumb side of the back of the forearm. Turning the palm downward is accomplished by using muscles located on the front of the forearm. Forearms are also the trademark of exceptional athletes of most throwing sports—baseball, football, and so on.

CHAPTER 7
PURE HARD LIFTS

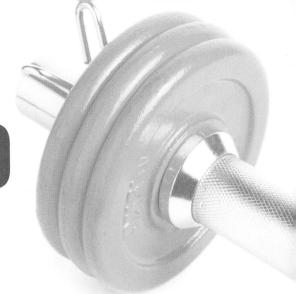

The core lifts are considered your basic movements: the Squat, Bench Press, Military Press, and the Deadlift. These are the only exercises you'll ever need, really, because they form the foundation of all other exercises. If worked hard enough for long periods of time, they'll turn you into a mountain of muscle.

■ ■ ■

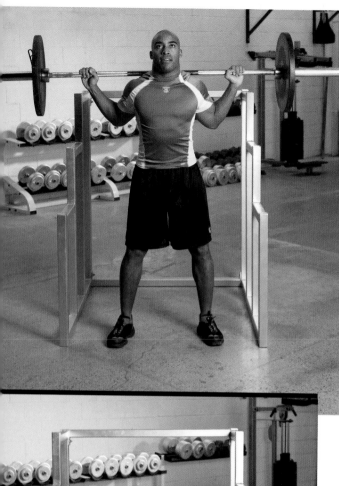

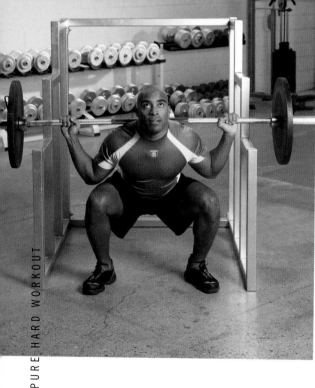

SQUAT

MUSCLE GROUP: all leg muscles and lower back

SETUP:

Grip a barbell in a squat rack with both hands. The distance between your hands should be about 6 inches wider than your shoulders.

Pull back your shoulders to form a ridge along your upper back, then duck under the bar and rest the weight on this ridge—not on your neck.

Push the weight from the rack by standing fully erect. Step back until you're clear of the rack supports and stand with your feet shoulder-width apart to provide steady balance and a proper position for the squat.

STEP ONE: Keep your shoulders tight and your eyes focused straight ahead as you push your hips back and lower yourself (as if sitting in a chair) until your upper thighs are parallel to the floor.

STEP TWO: Push the weight back up. When you arrive at your sticking point—where the maneuver becomes difficult for you—forcefully exhale. Ascend with your torso straight, not leaning too far forward.

When performing a Squat, focus on using the biggest, most powerful muscles of your thighs, hips, and buttocks. Taller men should place their feet beyond the width of their shoulders, with their toes pointing out. Squatting will be easier and more productive this way.

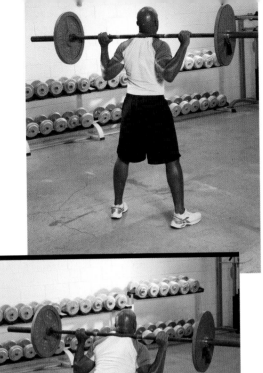

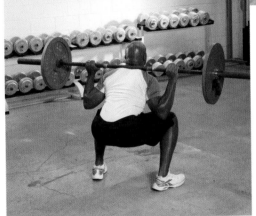

Tiki Tip: The Squat is the single most effective leg exercise ever conceived. If you learn how to squat correctly it will quickly become second nature for you and you most assuredly will reap the most benefits from the king of exercises.

KEYS TO SQUATTING

When squatting massive amounts of weight, keep these things in mind:

- A wide foot stance will give you better balance.
- Breathe deeply before you descend into the Squat.
- Resist exhaling until you're almost standing erect, then exhale forcefully.
- Always keep your head facing straight ahead, and your back flat. (Rounding your back can cause injuries.)
- Add weight to the bar whenever you can.
- Make sure you descend all the way—if you don't go down until your upper legs are parallel to the floor, it doesn't count. Lots of guys pile on the weight and then only squat halfway—don't be one of these guys.

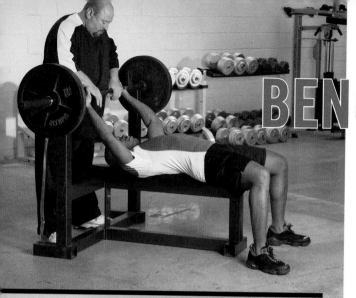

BENCH PRESS

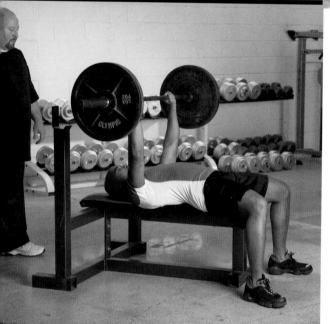

MUSCLE GROUP: pectorals, shoulder muscles, triceps, and upper and lower back

SETUP:

Lie on a bench with a rack for pressing. Place your feet flat on the floor and 18 to 24 inches apart for support.

Take a comfortable grip on the barbell. Your hands should be roughly shoulder-width apart. For safety and better control of the barbell, wrap your thumbs around the bar.

STEP ONE: Bring the barbell off the rack upright to arm's length. Use a spotter to help you get the bar out of the rack, if you want to. Lower your arms until they are at a ninety-degree angle, as you take a deep breath. The barbell should touch the center of the chest just above your nipples.

STEP TWO: Forcefully push the barbell back up, exhaling as you extend your arms.

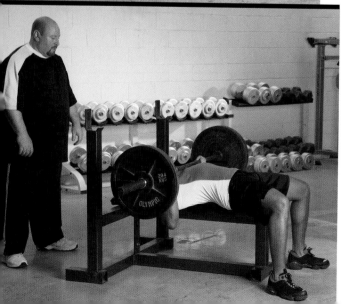

Some lifters arch their backs when bench-pressing, but this requires flexibility. People who do this sometimes develop lower-back pain if they're not set up properly. Always try

to pull your shoulder blades back before you press, to use the lats as a launching pad. The bar should touch your chest between presses. Use a spotter or spotters, if available.

Maximum width of your grip on the bar should be 32 inches. The closer together your hands are, the farther the bar has to travel, but this will help you develop your triceps and middle chest. The shorter your arms, the shorter the Bench Press stroke will be. There isn't much you can do about the length of your arms, although if you have exceptionally long arms you can try a wider grip to help cut down on the distance.

The 32-inch grip, however, does pose certain problems for people who can't refrain from using maximum weights in their training. This grip can and has caused shoulder strains and pectoral tears. If you feel shoulder pain with a wider grip, move your hands in a bit.

The medium grip (24 to 27 inches apart) should be used by those of you who are using remarkable poundage. This grip will give you the greatest explosion coming off the chest, but the lock-out is difficult. The lock-out will force you to use only triceps strength when finishing the lift. Ultimately, though, it's best to experiment with your grip to see which one best fits your individual needs.

Trying to bench heavy weight always involves the risk of injuries such as pectoral pulls, or shoulder and triceps tears. Your tendons and ligaments, in particular, are being asked to lift much more than they used to. It's crucial to utilize capable spotters. They can help you take the weight off the rack and save you if you get stuck during the lift. It's never recommended that you train alone. If you must, consider using a power rack so you can bench-press heavy weight in relative safety.

Tiki Tip: Plant your feet on the floor like two oak trees for stability. Make sure your eyes look up under the bar, and your forehead is beyond the barbell so that you don't hit the uprights while pressing the weight.

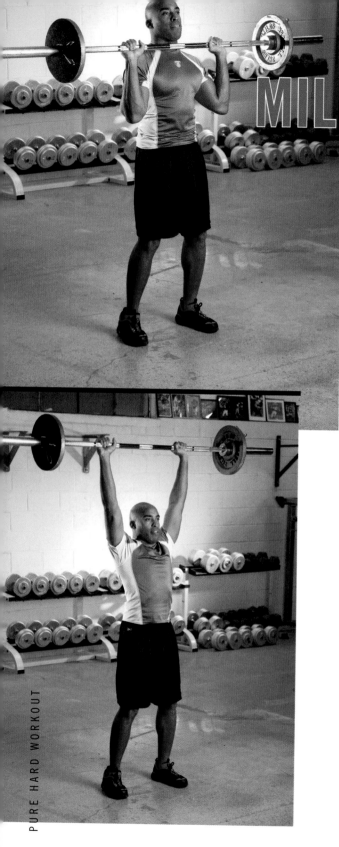

MILITARY PRESS

MUSCLE GROUP: deltoids, triceps, and trapezius

SETUP:

Stand with your feet 18 to 24 inches apart.

Grip a shoulder-high barbell on a rack so that your hands are each 3 to 5 inches wider than your shoulders.

STEP ONE: Lift the barbell off the stand (or rack) and lower it to the front of your shoulders.

STEP TWO: Press the weight straight and completely up.

Tiki Tip: On the descent, bring down the weight in a straight line. If you're flexible enough it should just touch your upper chest.

DEADLIFT

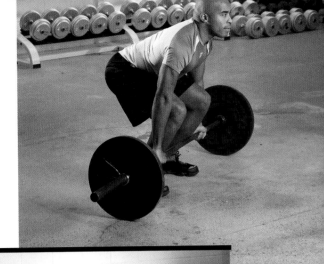

MUSCLE GROUP: all the pulling muscles of the body

Note: There are two distinct styles of the Deadlift. Both involve pulling a barbell from the floor, and both will make you a monster. We've outlined each of them here. Beginners will likely want to start with the bent-leg style (A) because it decreases the chance of injury and will give you a great feel for the movement. However, the rounded-back style (B) will allow you to move more total weight, and really pack muscle onto your back. Most record-setting deadlifts are done with style B.

STYLE A

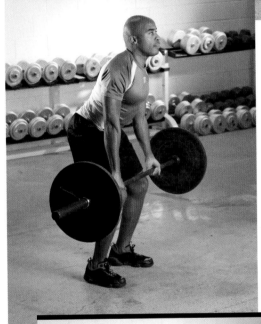

SETUP:

Place the barbell on the floor in front of your feet. Your feet should be shoulder-width apart and pointed slightly outward.

Squat down and grasp the bar tightly just outside your legs. As you squat down, the bar should just touch your shins and your knees should be over your toes. For added grip strength, you might want to use a mixed grip—your dominant hand over-hand and your other hand underhand.

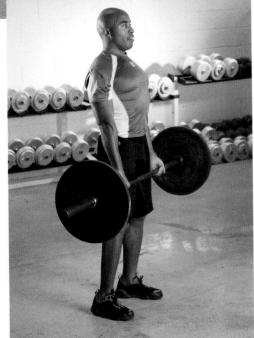

STEP ONE: Pull the barbell up while standing erect. Initiate the pull with your legs, and keep your back straight throughout the movement. The bar should be in contact with your legs throughout the movement, and at the very top pull back your shoulders to "lock out" the lift.

STYLE B

SETUP:

Place the barbell on the floor in front of your feet. Your feet should be shoulder-width apart and pointed slightly outward.

Grasp the bar tightly just outside your legs, using a mixed grip. There should be a slight roundness to your back, and a slight bend to your knees.

STEP ONE: Pull the barbell up while standing erect. Get the weight moving with your legs, but use your back muscles to continue the motion. You might find that you "hitch," or lose momentum, during the lift. Just keep pulling with all you've got. As with style A, the bar should be in contact with your legs throughout the movement, and you should pull back your shoulders to "lock out" the lift.

Tiki Tip: If your grip strength is preventing you from moving more weight in the Deadlift, you can use wrist straps. Keep in mind that these won't make your wrists and forearms any stronger, though.

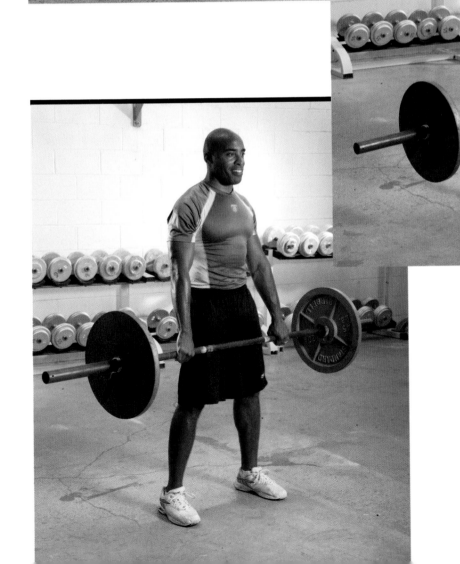

CHAPTER 8
VARIATIONS OF THE CORE LIFTS

This chapter demonstrates variations of the core lifts which are all good movements for building size and strength in specific body parts. For instance, the Incline Bench Press is great for building upper-chest size and power. For variety you can occasionally substitute dumbbells instead of always using a barbell.

■   ■   ■

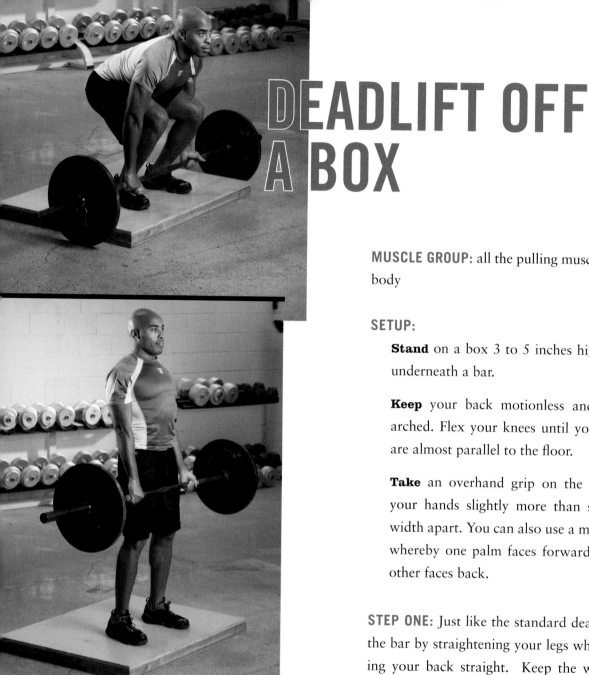

DEADLIFT OFF A BOX

MUSCLE GROUP: all the pulling muscles of the body

SETUP:

Stand on a box 3 to 5 inches high set up underneath a bar.

Keep your back motionless and a little arched. Flex your knees until your thighs are almost parallel to the floor.

Take an overhand grip on the bar with your hands slightly more than shoulder-width apart. You can also use a mixed grip whereby one palm faces forward and the other faces back.

STEP ONE: Just like the standard deadlift, lift the bar by straightening your legs while keeping your back straight. Keep the weight as close to your body as possible.

STEP TWO: Return the weight to the floor making sure you do not hyperextend or arch your back.

Tiki Tip: If your gym doesn't have a box for deadlifting, you can stand on top of two weight plates.

STIFF-LEGGED DEADLIFT

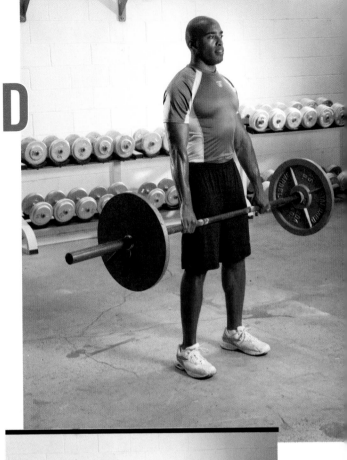

MUSCLE GROUP: hamstrings and lower back

SETUP:

Take a barbell off a rack set up at waist level, using an overhand grip just outside your shoulders (the rack is omitted in the photos to better illustrate the movement).

STEP ONE: Bend at the waist, keeping the barbell as close as possible to your legs and making sure not to arch your back. Stop just short of the floor, when your back is parallel to the ground.

STEP TWO: Exhale as you pull the weight back up to the starting position, making sure you keep your back straight. Your knees don't bend, but they shouldn't be completely locked out, either.

Tiki Tip: You should really feel this in your hamstrings, not in your back. You can hurt yourself if you arch your back while doing this, so make sure it stays straight.

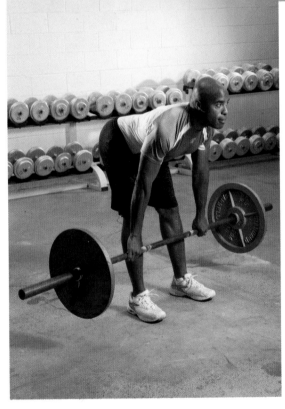

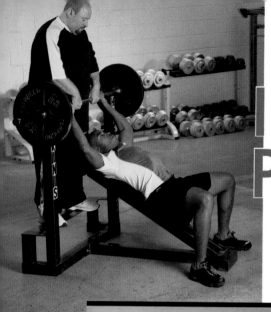

INCLINE BENCH PRESS

MUSCLE GROUP: pectorals

SETUP:

Lie on a forty-five-degree inclined bench with a rack for pressing.

Grip the barbell. The distance between your hands on the bar should be slightly wider than your shoulders. Your grip should be similar to the one you use for the Bench Press.

STEP ONE: Take the bar from the rack with a spotter's help if needed, and lower it to within 2 to 3 inches of your chin. Inhale deeply as the weight is lowered.

STEP TWO: Press the bar all the way up, exhaling as you do so.

Tiki Tip: Press the weight from right under your chin; this ensures that you're working the upper-chest muscles. The bar should just hit your upper chest. Using a spotter is a good idea, especially to assist with moving the bar on and off the rack.

DECLINE BENCH PRESS

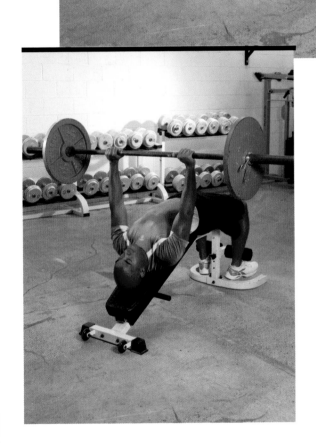

MUSCLE GROUP: pectorals and triceps

SETUP:

Lie on a decline bench that includes a rack for pressing (the rack is omitted here).

Grip the barbell and take it from the rack. The distance between your hands on the bar should be slightly wider than your shoulders. Your grip should be similar to the one you use for the Bench Press.

STEP ONE: Bring the barbell toward your chest, to within 2 or 3 inches of your nipples.

STEP TWO: Push the bar up over your chest as you straighten your arms. A slight 1- to 3-second pause is recommended when the bar is at its lowest point, but don't bounce the barbell; just use pure pectoral power.

Tiki Tip: You should vary your grip from 24 to 32 inches to see which one is most comfortable and most productive. This exercise is particularly great for lower pectoral development.

CLOSE-GRIP BENCH PRESS

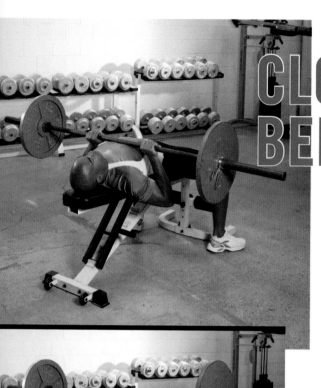

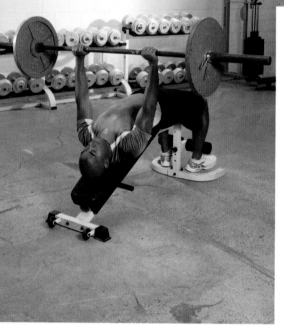

MUSCLE GROUP: pectorals and triceps

SETUP:

Lie on your back on a flat bench with a rack for pressing (the rack is omitted here).

Take an overhand grip on the barbell with your hands from 6 to 24 inches apart, depending on your wrist flexibility. Your hands should definitely be closer together than the grip you use for the standard bench press.

Take the barbell from the rack and hold it straight overhead.

STEP ONE: Inhale and slowly lower the barbell until it reaches your chest, with your elbows extending out.

STEP TWO: Press the barbell upward, exhaling as you complete the movement.

Tiki Tip: As with any bench press, it's a good idea to have a spotter for this exercise. The closer your hands are together, the more this exercise will blast your triceps.

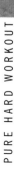

SEATED PRESS

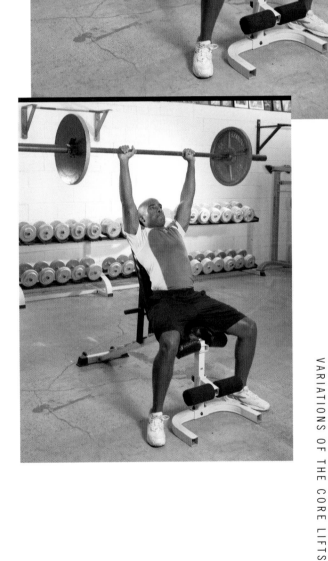

MUSCLE GROUP: deltoids, upper pectorals, traps, triceps

SETUP:

Sit on an eighty-degree incline bench situated underneath a barbell in a rack (the rack is omitted here to better illustrate the exercise).

Grab the barbell with an overhand grip just outside your shoulders and remove it from the rack, letting it just touch your upper chest.

STEP ONE: Inhale, then press the barbell straight up, exhaling at the top of the movement.

STEP TWO: Slowly return to the starting position.

Tiki Tip: You'll be able to move more weight in the Seated Press than the Military Press because sitting down takes the strain off your lower back as you press.

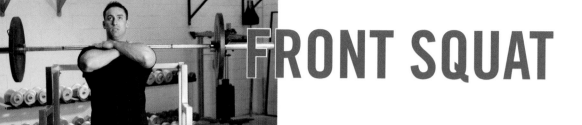

FRONT SQUAT

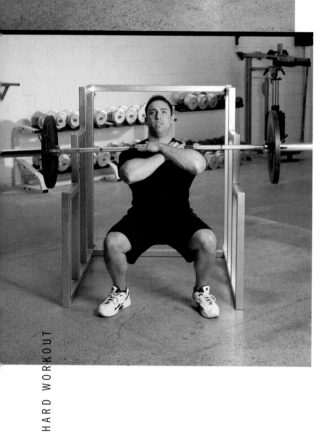

MUSCLE GROUP: quadriceps, hamstrings, abdominals, and lower back

SETUP:

Position a barbell in a rack at the same height you'd use for a standard squat.

Place the barbell across the front of your upper chest, forming a ridge for it to rest on by extending your arms out straight ahead.

Bend your elbows, cross your arms, and rest your hands across the top of the bar to steady it as you take it out of the rack.

STEP ONE: Squat down, just as with the standard squat, inhaling as you do so.

STEP TWO: Push the weight back up as you exhale.

(Pictured is Joe's son Eric. Strength runs in the family.)

Tiki Tip: This one can be a little bit tricky, so start out with light weight. Because of the placement of the bar, this one will tax you differently than the standard squat.

DUMBBELL FLY

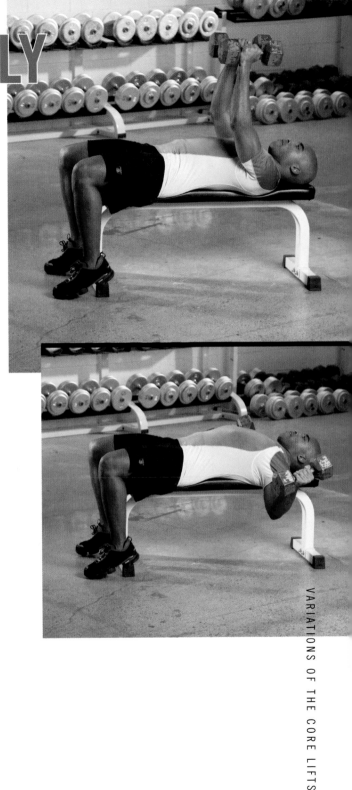

MUSCLE GROUP: pectorals

SETUP:

Lie flat on your back on a bench.

Start with a pair of dumbbells held at arm's length over your chest.

Bend your arms slightly to take pressure off your elbows.

STEP ONE: Lower the weights out to your sides as far as you can while inhaling as much air as possible.

STEP TWO: Raise your arms back to the start position, exhaling and tensing your chest muscles as you do. You will be making a wide circle with the dumbbells.

Tiki Tip: Be sure to get a full stretch by lowering the dumbbells as far as possible on each repetition. Some guys use dumbbells that are too heavy and make it into a dumbbell-pressing movement, but we're not looking for that.

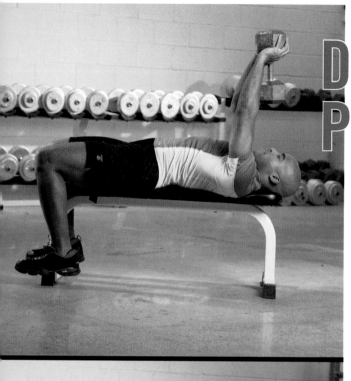

DUMBBELL PULLOVER

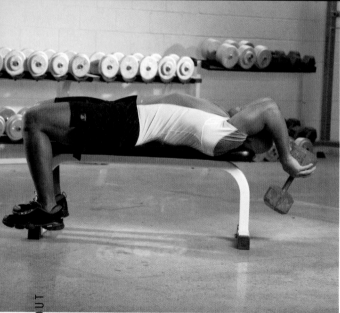

MUSCLE GROUP: pectorals, lats, and abs

SETUP:

Lie on your back on a bench.

Flatten your hands against the inside of one end of a dumbbell.

Hold the dumbbell at arm's length over your chest.

STEP ONE: Lower the dumbbell while inhaling deeply until the end you're holding is in line with your head.

STEP TWO: Exhale as you return the weight to starting position, making sure you don't clock yourself with the weight.

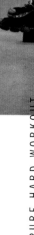

Tiki Tip: Inhale as deeply as possible. Force all the air you can into your lungs, and keep your chest expanded even after you exhale.

DUMBBELL ONE-ARM ROW

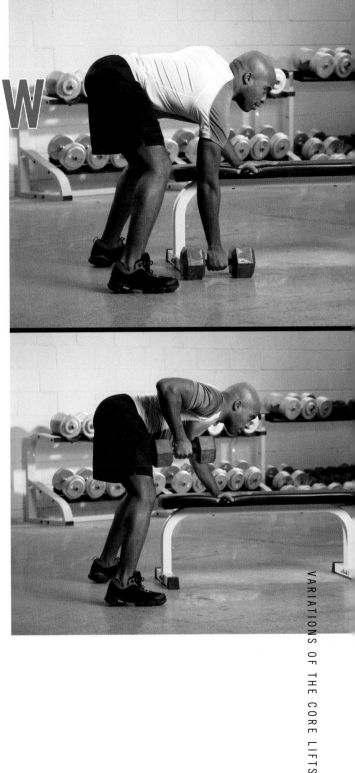

MUSCLE GROUP: lats, biceps, and forearms

SETUP:

Place one hand and one knee on a bench, or just place one hand on a bench, whichever is more comfortable.

Lean over with the opposite arm and grab a dumbbell.

STEP ONE: Pull the dumbbell into the side of your body toward your armpit.

STEP TWO: Slowly lower the dumbbell. Keep your core stationary, moving just your arm.

Tiki Tip: If the dumbbell gets too heavy with one knee on the bench, keep both feet on the floor and instead straddle the bench. More weight can be used this way, and you won't lose your balance. Find a steady rhythm, and row with conviction.

VARIATIONS OF THE CORE LIFTS

73

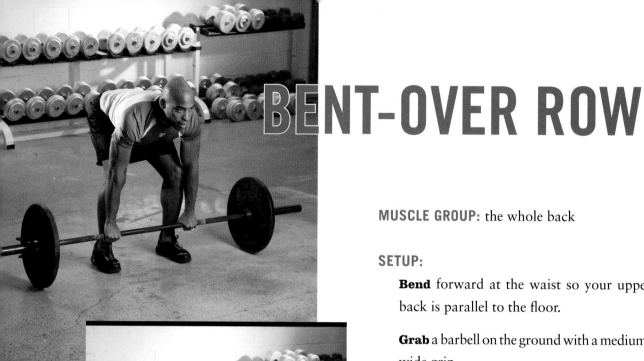

BENT-OVER ROW

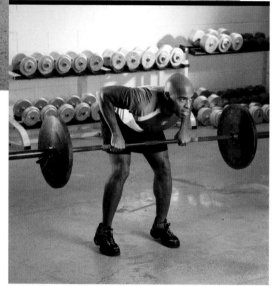

MUSCLE GROUP: the whole back

SETUP:

Bend forward at the waist so your upper back is parallel to the floor.

Grab a barbell on the ground with a medium-wide grip.

Keep your knees slightly bent.

STEP ONE: Pull the bar up until it touches your stomach.

STEP TWO: Lower it slowly until your arms are fully extended, but don't let the bar return to the ground.

Use an overhand grip, but occasionally mix in the underhand grip. A good technique is to use the same grip width for your barbell rows as you would the Bench Press. Your back should always remain flat throughout the movement. Some people pick up the bar and do only a quarter of the motion, invariably hurting their backs. Don't worry about the amount of weight you're lifting; get the form down first, and as you get stronger, you'll be able to increase the weight.

Tiki Tip: Make your back muscles do all the work. Don't tense the biceps as you pull upward. Think of the hands and arms as hooks pulling the bar to your lower stomach. If you pull it to your chest, your elbows can't move back far enough to complete the move.

CHIN-UP

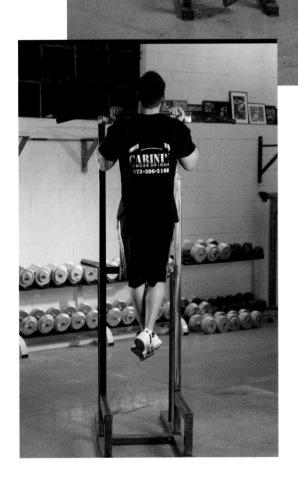

MUSCLE GROUP: the whole back

SETUP:

Hang from the bar with an underhand grip.

STEP ONE: Pull yourself up until your chin is over the bar.

STEP TWO: Lower yourself slowly. Keep your legs slightly bent. Don't make any cheating movements with your waist or hips.

Tiki Tip: To avoid swaying as you pull yourself up, try crossing your legs. When you get strong enough to do, say, 10 repetitions on your own, add additional weight with a weight belt to make your Chin-ups tougher.

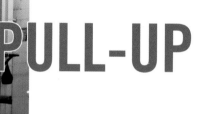

PULL-UP

MUSCLE GROUP: the whole back

SETUP:

Hang from the bar with a wide overhand grip.

STEP ONE: Take a breath and pull yourself upward until your eyes are above the level of the bar, exhaling as you complete the movement.

STEP TWO: Lower yourself slowly, keeping your weight under control.

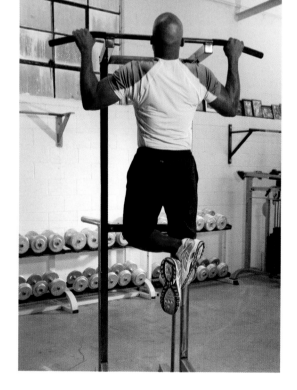

Tiki Tip: The farther apart your hands are, the harder this exercise will be.

DIP

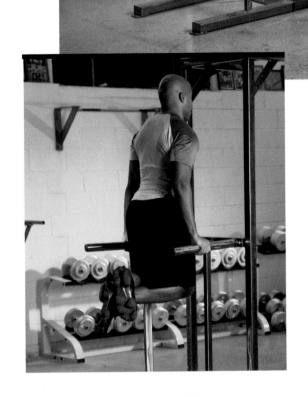

MUSCLE GROUP: delts, triceps, and pecs

SETUP:

Hop onto the dipping station.

Grab the hand grips with your hands at waist level and the distance between them slightly wider than your shoulder width.

Push yourself up and lift up your legs, leaving the ground. Remain in this position, holding your body weight.

STEP ONE: Lower your body as slowly and as low as you can—try to touch your front shoulders to the bars.

STEP TWO: Press your body weight up again. Keep your legs bent.

Tiki Tip: Look directly ahead during the movements and try to keep your body as straight as possible. Go up and down evenly but slowly. If you lean forward too much, this maneuver becomes a strict pectoral exercise. Leaning backward will work your triceps more. When you become strong on body-weight Dips, then you can add additional weight with weight belts.

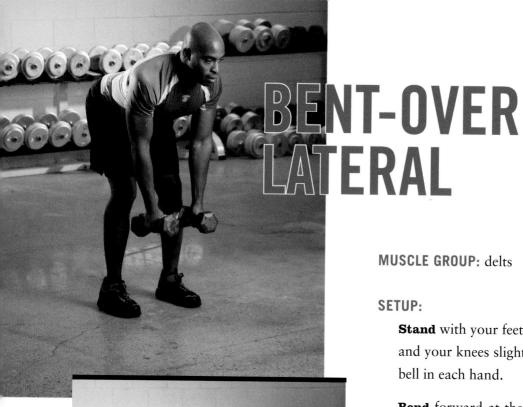

BENT-OVER LATERAL

MUSCLE GROUP: delts

SETUP:

Stand with your feet shoulder-width apart and your knees slightly bent with a dumbbell in each hand.

Bend forward at the waist and keep your back straight.

Hold the dumbbells with your elbows slightly bent.

STEP ONE: Raise the dumbbells to your sides and hold, exhaling as you complete the movement.

STEP TWO: Return to the starting position.

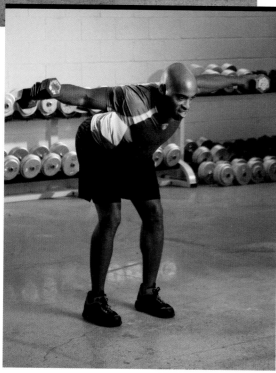

Tiki Tip: It's important to do rear-deltoid exercises using good form and without jerking the body up and down. Slow, controlled reps work best.

LATERAL RAISE

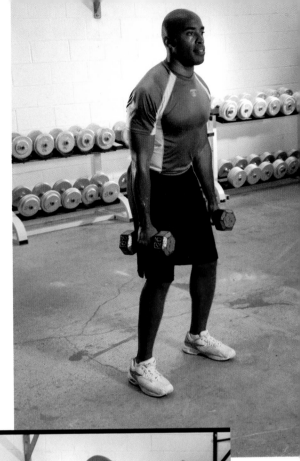

MUSCLE GROUP: delts

SETUP:

    Stand with a dumbbell in each hand with an overhand grip.

    Hold the dumbbells at your side with a slight bend in your elbows.

STEP ONE: Lift the dumbbells up just higher than your shoulders.

STEP TWO: Return to the starting position.

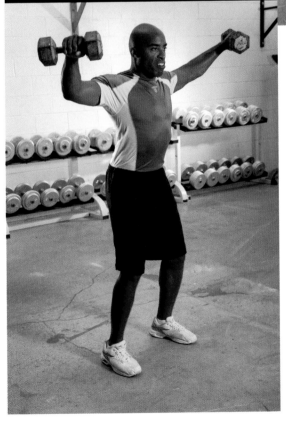

Tiki Tip: If you want to make this a little more challenging, try turning your wrists so your thumbs point up while you execute the movement. This will really work your shoulders.

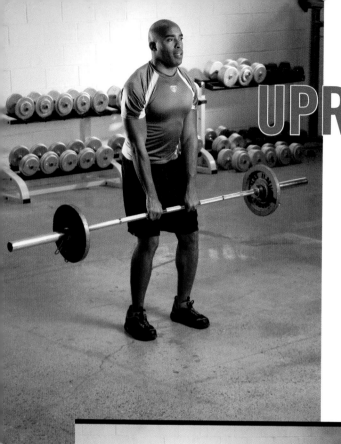

UPRIGHT ROW

MUSCLE GROUP: delts and upper back

SETUP:

Stand with a barbell in front of your thighs.

Hold bar with an overhand grip, your hands 10 to 18 inches apart on the bar, depending on your size.

STEP ONE: Pull the weight toward your upper chest with your arms bent and elbows held high.

STEP TWO: Return the weight to the starting position, resisting it on the way down.

Tiki Tip: Keep the weight close to your body; don't let it drift out in front of you.

SHRUG

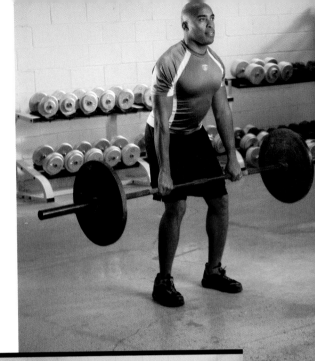

MUSCLE GROUP: traps (also improves your grip when you're holding heavy weights)

SETUP:

Place a barbell on a rack (omitted here to make picture clearer) at mid-thigh level.

Grip with your hands 32 inches apart.

Keep your arms straight as you remove the bar from the rack.

STEP ONE: Shrug your shoulders up until you can't shrug them any higher, keeping your arms straight. Try to get your traps to touch your ears.

STEP TWO: Slowly lower your shoulders.

Powerlifters use Shrugs with heavy weights because it helps them build "lock-out" power in deadlifting. Lock-out power is necessary to complete a deadlift as you kick your hips through the sticking point where the lift is the toughest. The workout continues from there to develop more strength throughout the lift.

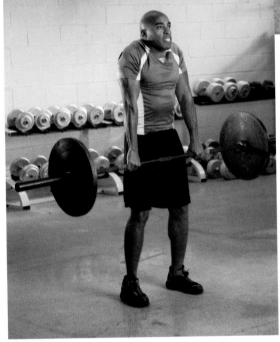

Tiki Tip: When heavy weights are used, you can use lifting straps to help you grip. You can also perform this lift with dumbbells.

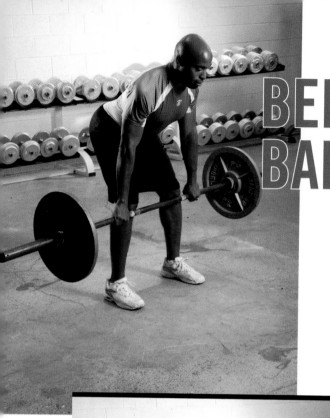

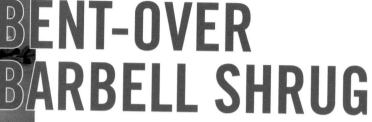

BENT-OVER BARBELL SHRUG

MUSCLE GROUP: upper back, traps

SETUP:

Hold a barbell as with the standard shrug.

Bend forward at the waist so your upper back is parallel to the floor.

Keep your knees bent.

STEP ONE: Shrug your shoulders upward, and then roll them slightly backward and finish the movement by arching your back.

STEP TWO: Slowly return to the starting position.

Tiki Tip: One variation is to use a close grip with your knuckles up. Another is to grip the barbell underhanded, which works the back muscles. Still another is to perform a full rotating motion. This can become an incredibly strenuous exercise.

STANDING BARBELL CURL

MUSCLE GROUP: biceps

SETUP:

Stand with a barbell, your hands shoulder-width apart on the bar using an underhand grip.

Let the bar just rest against your thighs.

STEP ONE: Keep your back in its natural position, as you curl the barbell using only biceps.

STEP TWO: Slowly lower the bar along the same pathway. Your upper arms should remain in the same position throughout the exercise.

Tiki Tip: Keep your upper arms next to your sides. Definitely do not swing the weight when curling; using momentum like this is considered cheating, and won't make you stronger.

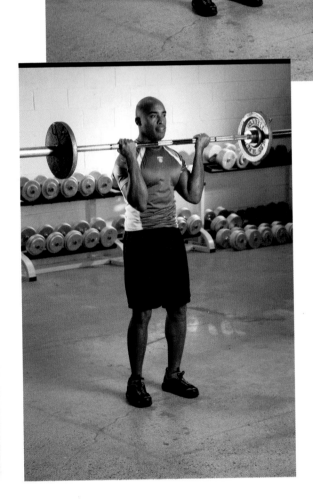

GOOD MORNING

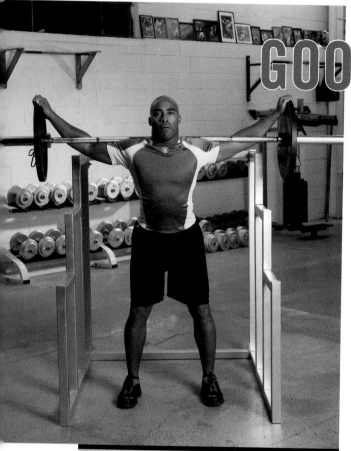

MUSCLE GROUP: lower back, hamstrings, and abdominals

SETUP:

Using straight legs, stand with your feet slightly apart.

Place a barbell on your back as if you were going to execute a Squat.

Keep your knees slightly bent.

STEP ONE: Bend at the waist as far as you can, until your upper body is parallel to the floor.

STEP TWO: Return to starting position, exhaling and keeping your back straight.

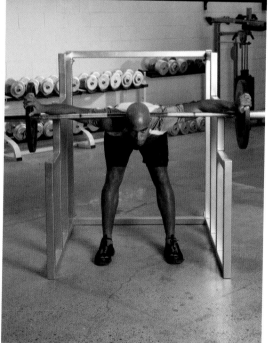

Tiki Tip: Tiki prefers to keep his hands on the weight plates, but you can keep them in the standard squat position if it's more comfortable for you.

BACK EXTENSION (HYPEREXTENSION)

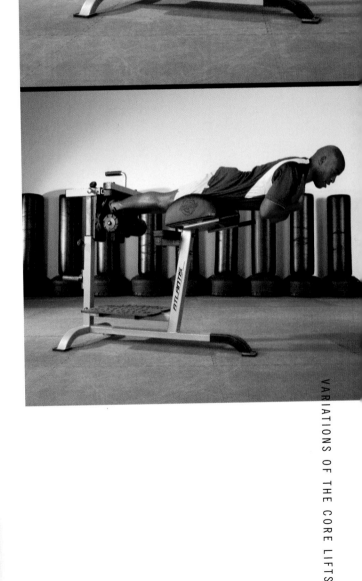

MUSCLE GROUP: butt and hamstrings

SETUP:

Lie facedown on a Roman chair with the ankle supports properly adjusted and your hips on the support pads.

Place your hands behind your head or on your chest.

Lower your head until your upper body is at a ninety-degree angle to your lower body.

STEP ONE: Raise your upper body until it's slightly above your lower body and parallel to the floor.

STEP TWO: Return to the starting position.

Tiki Tip: Be sure to keep your back arched to reduce the chance of injury.

POWER CLEAN

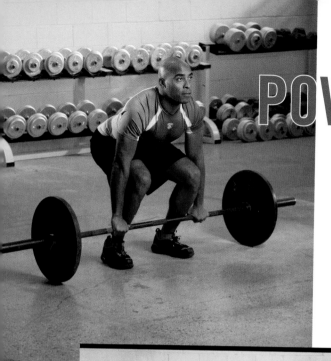

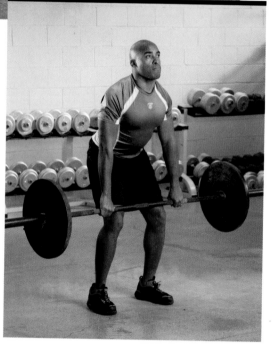

MUSCLE GROUP: almost everything

SETUP:

> **Get** into the Deadlift position: Stand with your feet under a barbell, slightly wider than your shoulders. Bend forward, hands outside of your knees, keeping your back parallel to the floor, and grab the bar with an overhand grip.

STEP ONE: The idea is to straighten out your body in one motion and end up with the bar at your shoulders. To begin the movement, use your legs and hips to pull the weight off the ground.

STEP TWO: You actually want to pull the bar as high as possible, then dip under it as you catch it.

Tiki Tip: Learn good technique and think of pulling the bar with speed, but at all times keep the bar as close to your body as possible. Learn to pull with your legs, back, and traps, but not with your arms. Be sure to master this technique with light weight before you move on to heavy poundage.

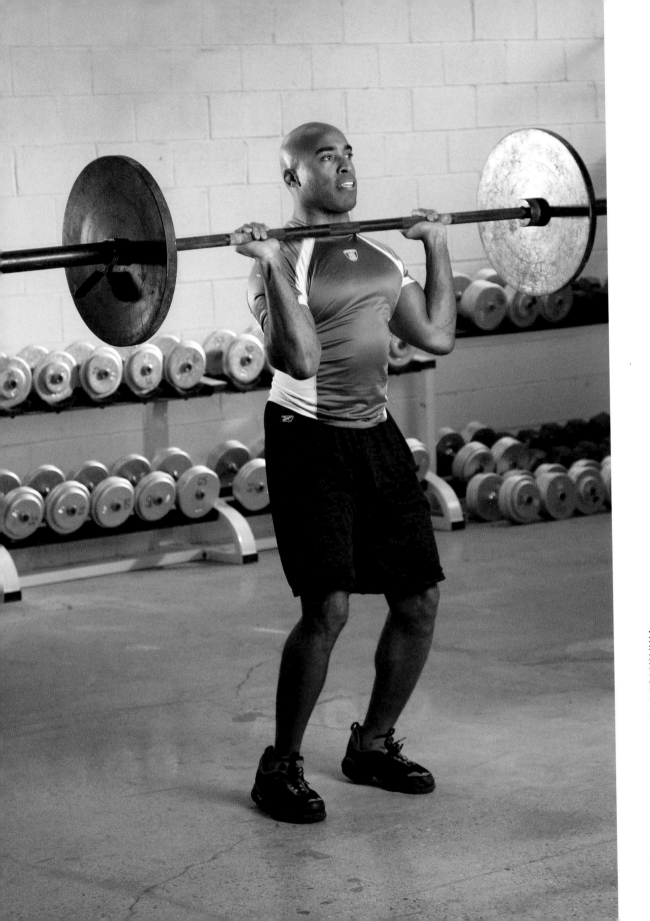

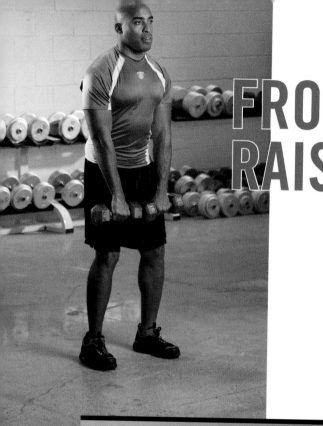

FRONT DUMBBELL RAISE

MUSCLE GROUP: shoulders

SETUP:

Stand with a dumbbell in each hand using an overhand grip. Your arms should be straight, and the dumbbells in front of your thighs.

STEP ONE: Keeping your arms straight, bring the dumbbells to just above shoulder height.

STEP TWO: Lower your arms back to starting position, slowly and under control.

Tiki Tip: Some people like to do both arms at the same time; others like to alternate one arm, and then the other. A slight bend at the knees is acceptable, and using a little momentum is okay especially when you build up to higher poundage.

STANDING TRICEPS EXTENSION

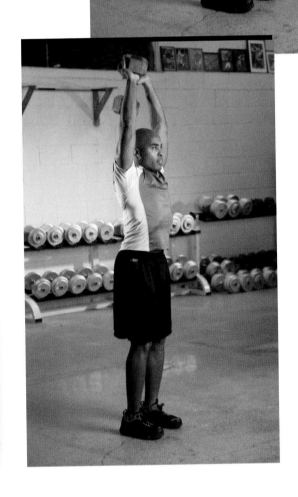

MUSCLE GROUP: triceps

SETUP:

Stand with a dumbbell gripped vertically in both hands, one fist above the other on the bar.

Place the dumbbell behind your head at the back of your neck, your elbows pointing to the ceiling. Most people put both palms flat against the plate of the dumbbell.

STEP ONE: Lift the dumbbell straight over your head, holding your upper arms against your ears.

STEP TWO: Drop the weight slowly down behind your neck.

Tiki Tip: Only your forearms should move. The upper arms should remain against the sides of your head and not move at all. Instead of dumbbells, you can also use a barbell or EZ curl bar. Both are extremely effective.

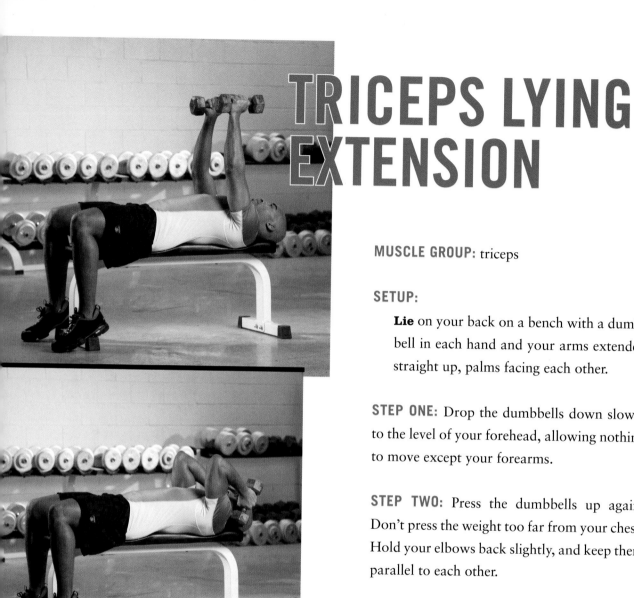

TRICEPS LYING EXTENSION

MUSCLE GROUP: triceps

SETUP:

> **Lie** on your back on a bench with a dumbbell in each hand and your arms extended straight up, palms facing each other.

STEP ONE: Drop the dumbbells down slowly to the level of your forehead, allowing nothing to move except your forearms.

STEP TWO: Press the dumbbells up again. Don't press the weight too far from your chest. Hold your elbows back slightly, and keep them parallel to each other.

Tiki Tip: Some lifters like to do these lying on the floor with someone spotting them. If you're doing this by yourself, don't drop the weight on your head.

TRICEPS DUMBBELL KICKBACK

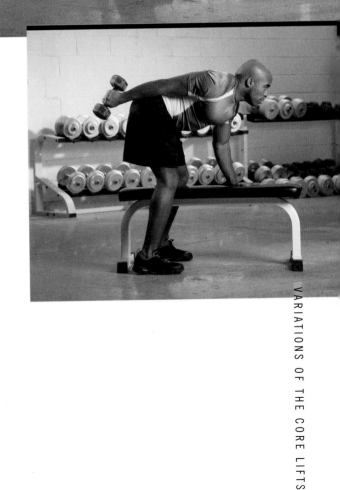

MUSCLE GROUP: triceps

SETUP:

> **Stand** with your knees slightly flexed and one hand on a bench, bending forward at the waist and keeping your back straight.

> **Hold** a dumbbell in your other hand with your elbow bent at a ninety-degree angle.

STEP ONE: Straighten your arm. Exhale as you complete the movement.

STEP TWO: Return to the starting position.

Tiki Tip: This exercise is excellent for the entire triceps.

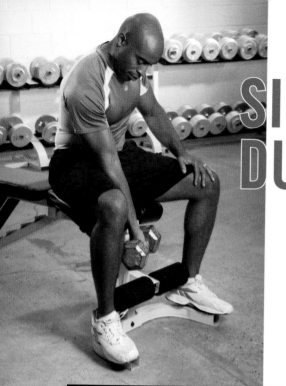

SITTING DUMBBELL CURL

MUSCLE GROUP: biceps

SETUP:

> **Sit** on a bench holding a dumbbell in one hand with your palm facing inward and your elbow braced against your inner thigh.

STEP ONE: Raise your arm, keeping your elbow in contact with your thigh.

STEP TWO: Lower your arm back to the start position.

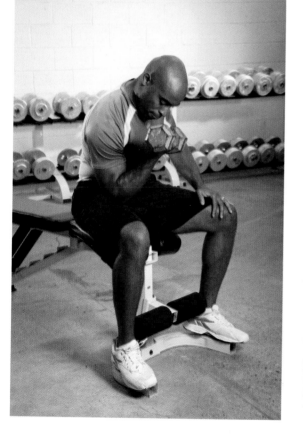

Tiki Tip: This exercise is excellent for emphasizing the biceps in all its actions. Again, don't swing the weight when curling; using momentum is considered cheating. This exercise is also referred to as the Concentration Curl, so concentrate!

INCLINE DUMBBELL CURL

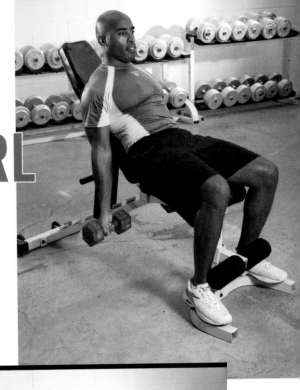

MUSCLE GROUP: biceps

SETUP:

Sit on a bench angled at forty-five degrees, holding a dumbbell in each hand with your palms up.

STEP ONE: Inhale, then curl the weight up. Raise your elbow at the top of the movement.

STEP TWO: Slowly return the weight to the starting position.

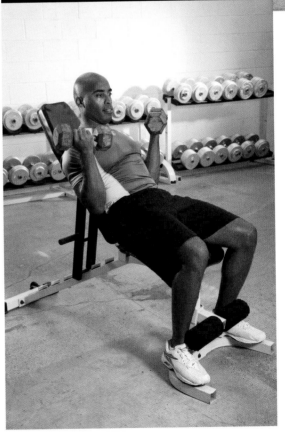

Tiki Tip: You can either curl both arms at the same time or alternate them. It comes down to personal preference.

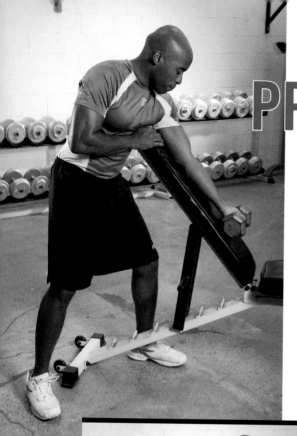

PREACHER CURL

MUSCLE GROUP: biceps

SETUP:

Stand behind an incline bench.

Grip a dumbbell in one hand and rest your upper arm against the bench.

STEP ONE: Raise the dumbbell as far as you can, as with a normal curl.

STEP TWO: Slowly lower the dumbbell until your arm is back resting against the bench.

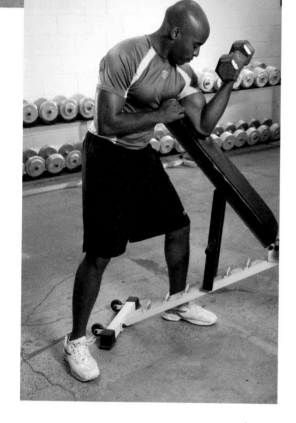

Tiki Tip: Many gyms have a Preacher Curl station, which you can use instead of an incline bench.

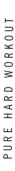

DUMBBELL HAMMER CURL

MUSCLE GROUP: biceps and forearms

SETUP:

Grasp a dumbbell in each hand with your palms facing inward.

STEP ONE: Curl the dumbbells to your shoulders. Exhale as you complete the movement.

STEP TWO: Slowly return the weights to the starting position.

Tiki Tip: I used this movement to build thickness in my biceps and forearms.

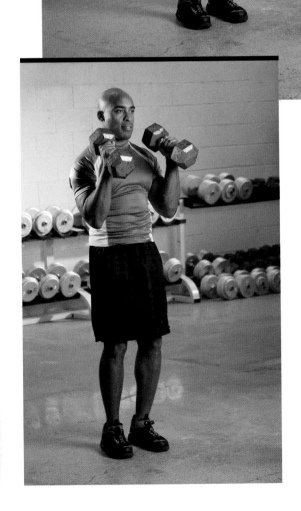

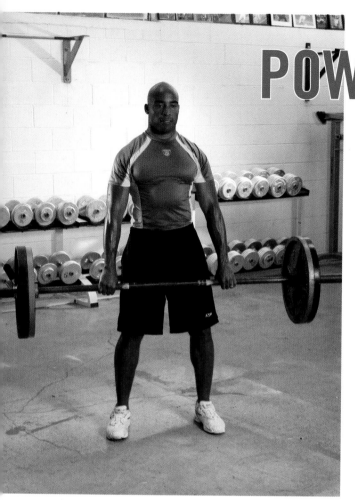

POWER HOLD

MUSCLE GROUP: forearms

SETUP:

Use a power rack and position the barbell an inch or two above the knees (rack not pictured here).

Grab the bar with an overhand grip.

STEP ONE: Take the weight from the rack and hold it as long as you can.

Tiki Tip: Keep your hands on the outside of the thighs and use the strength of your hands and fingers alone to hold the bar. A reverse grip with one hand facing forward and the other hand facing backward (the way a powerlifter holds the bar for Deadlifting) would be too easy. Be sure to hold the bar rather than leaning back and resting the bar on your upper thighs.

SEATED WRIST CURL

MUSCLE GROUP: wrists and forearms

SETUP:

Sit on a bench.

Rest the back of one forearm on your thigh. Your wrist should be hanging off your knees.

STEP ONE: Curl the weight up until your forearm is contracted.

STEP TWO: Let the weight down slowly, and then extend the weight down to your fingers and curl your wrist up again.

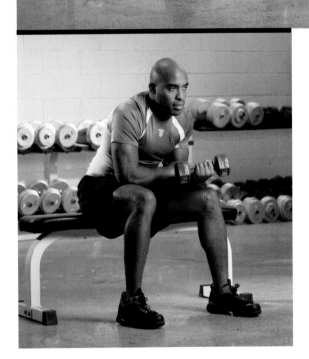

Tiki Tip: Try this with an overhand grip, too, for more complete forearm development.

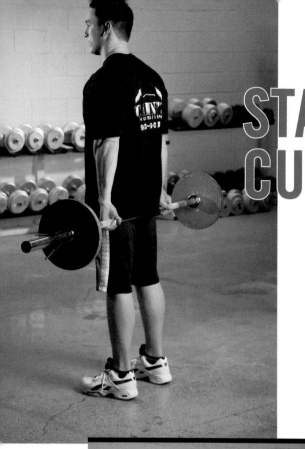

STANDING WRIST CURL

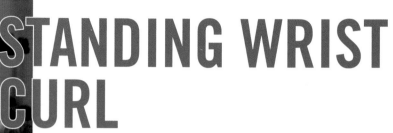

MUSCLE GROUP: wrists

SETUP:

Stand with the barbell behind you, preferably sitting on a rack (rack not pictured here). Your arms should be hanging straight down.

Grab the barbell using an underhand grip with your hands slightly wider than shoulder-width apart.

STEP ONE: Curl your wrists away from your body, bringing your hands up.

STEP TWO: Return the weight to the starting position.

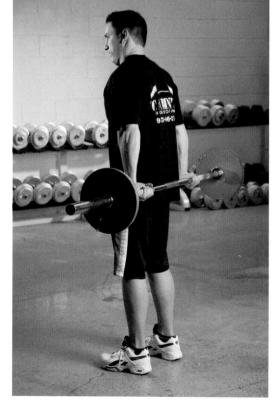

Tiki Tip: Vary your hand placement from narrow to wide for a more complete workout.

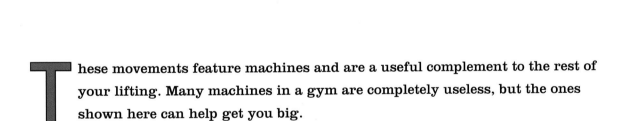

CHAPTER 9
ASSISTED
MOVEMENTS

These movements feature machines and are a useful complement to the rest of your lifting. Many machines in a gym are completely useless, but the ones shown here can help get you big.

■   ■   ■

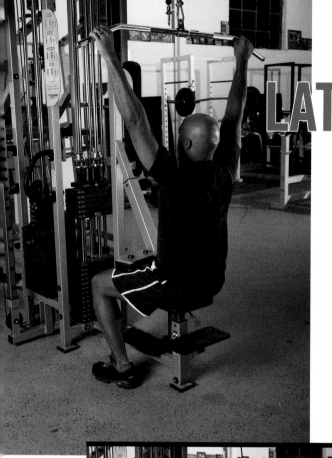

LAT PULLDOWN

MUSCLE GROUP: lats, biceps, and shoulders

SETUP:

Grasp the bar.

Sit with your upper body in an upright position, knees locked under the pad, leaning back slightly from the hips.

STEP ONE: Pull the bar down in front of your face and to your chest, and pause.

STEP TWO: Slowly release the bar to the starting position by straightening your arms.

Tiki Tip: You can do this exercise with an overhand, underhand, or mixed grip. Vary your hand placement to get a complete workout.

SHOULDER PRESS MACHINE

MUSCLE GROUP: delts, upper traps, triceps

SETUP:

Sit on the machine with your back straight and grasp the handles.

STEP ONE: Inhale, then press overhead without arching your back, exhaling as you lock out the weight.

STEP TWO: Return to the starting position.

Tiki Tip: You can work up to massive amounts of poundage on this exercise, as Joe demonstrates—those plates weigh 100 pounds each.

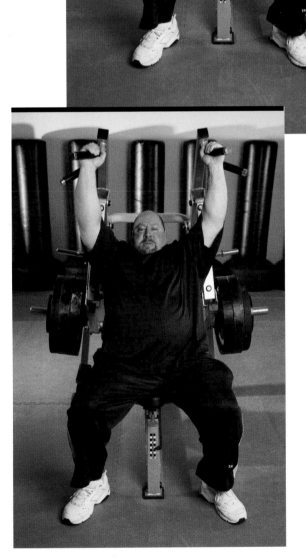

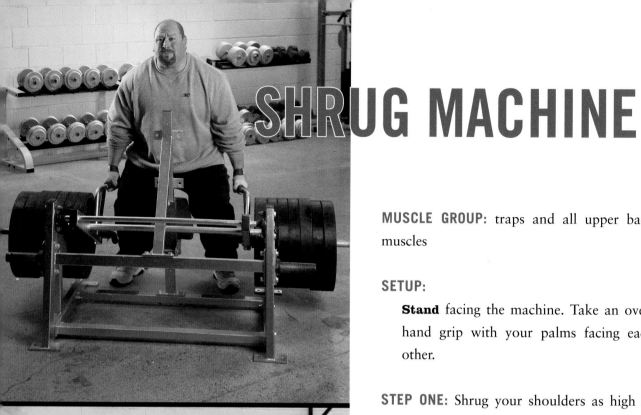

SHRUG MACHINE

MUSCLE GROUP: traps and all upper back muscles

SETUP:

Stand facing the machine. Take an overhand grip with your palms facing each other.

STEP ONE: Shrug your shoulders as high as you can, keeping your head back and your back straight.

STEP TWO: Return to the starting position.

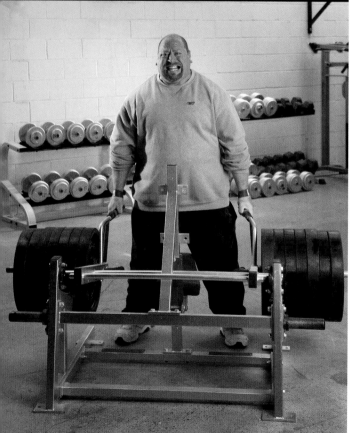

Tiki Tip: Like the shoulder press machine, you can move big weights safely with this apparatus. Just maybe not 1,400 pounds like Joe.

CABLE ROW

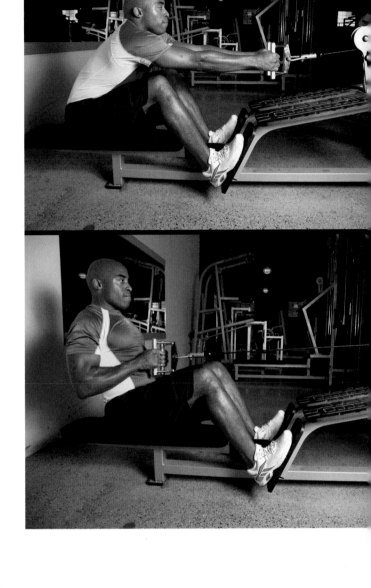

MUSCLE GROUP: lats, traps, and biceps

SETUP:

Sit on the bench, facing the machine.

Lean forward and grab the cable handle.

STEP ONE: Keeping knees slightly bent, pull the handle into your lower abdomen, and hold. Avoid leaning back too far.

STEP TWO: Slowly let the cable handle return to the starting position.

Tiki Tip: You can use a variety of handles, but the standard one is V-shaped, which allows you to pull your arms all the way back for a full range of movement. As always, good form is the most important thing to remember. Let your upper back and arms do all the work.

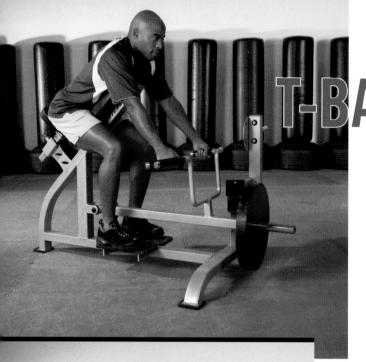

T-BAR ROW

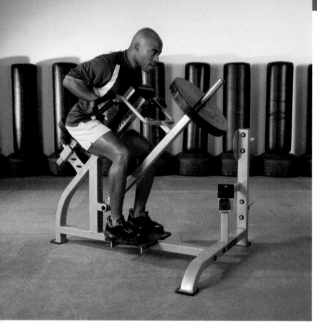

MUSCLE GROUP: lats

SETUP: The T-bar lies horizontally on the floor. One end of the bar is attached to the floor and the other is loose and ends in a short handle.

Straddle the central bar.

Lean your chest against the pad.

Take the innermost grip on the handles and pull the weight off its rack.

STEP ONE: Pull the T-bar up until your hands hit your chest. Keep your chest on the pad.

STEP TWO: Lower the weight back to its starting position.

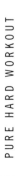
Tiki Tip: If you don't have access to a T-Bar Row, try to cobble one together by wedging one end of a barbell into a corner, putting weights on other edge, and then pulling it to your chest using a V-handle. Just don't jerk the weight and injure your lower back.

TRICEPS PUSHDOWN

MUSCLE GROUP: triceps

SETUP:

> **Hang** a rope handle from the cable weight stack.

> **Stand** facing the stack and grab the ends of the rope. If you use a heavy weight, lean slightly forward at the waist for more stability.

STEP ONE: Pull the rope down until it touches your thighs. Nothing should move except your forearms. Your upper body, legs, and upper arms should remain still.

STEP TWO: Hold the weight with your triceps for 2 seconds to feel the movement more intensely and then return to the starting position.

Tiki Tip: You can also perform this movement with a bar instead of a rope, but it will be a little easier.

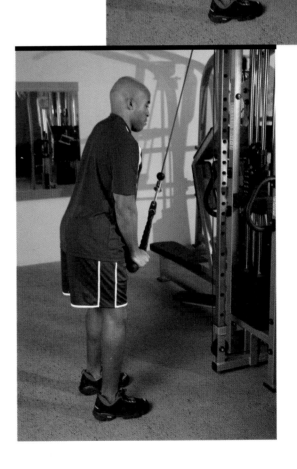

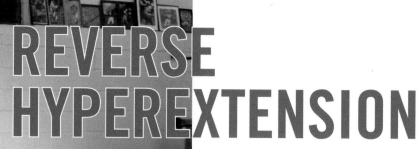

REVERSE HYPEREXTENSION

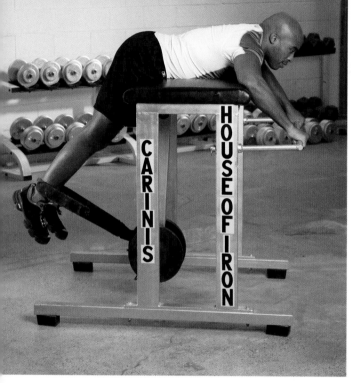

MUSCLE GROUP: spinal erectors, thighs, butt, and abs.

SETUP:

This is best done on a dedicated reverse-hyper apparatus, but you can also do it on a high box, a butt-and-hamstrings machine, or a back extension bench.

Lie on your stomach with your legs hanging down and the strap around your ankles.

STEP ONE: Forcibly raise your legs until they're parallel to the floor, keeping them straight.

STEP TWO: Return to the starting position, keeping tension on the strap.

Tiki Tip: High reps will give you a great lower-back pump.

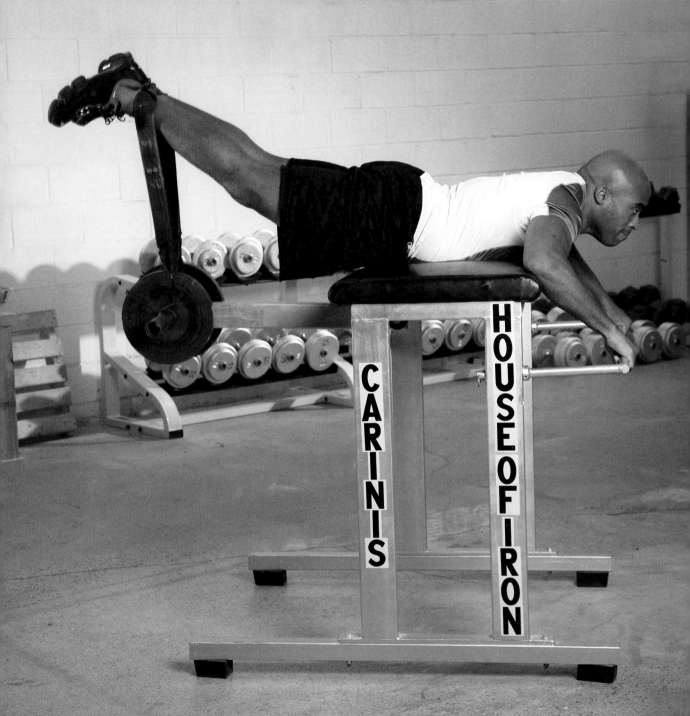

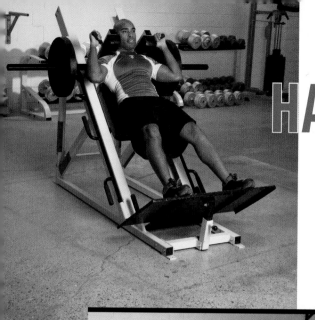

HACK SQUAT

MUSCLE GROUP: quads

SETUP:

Flex your knees and place your back against the padded surface.

Wedge your shoulders beneath the yokes attached to the machine and place your feet fairly close together. Most people prefer to grab the handles, too.

Inhale, rotate the stop handles to release the weight, and let the weight bend your legs into a deep squat.

STEP ONE: Push the weight back up to the starting position, exhaling as you do so. To protect your back from injury, be sure to contract your abdominals in order to avoid swinging your pelvis and spine.

STEP TWO: Inhale as you descend back into the squat.

When you've completed your set, push the weight back up to the top and lock the weight with the catch. Make sure the weight is locked before you try to step out from under it!

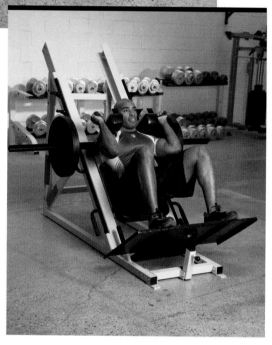

Tiki Tip: There is also a version of this machine in which you stand facing the weight. It works essentially the same way.

LEG PRESS

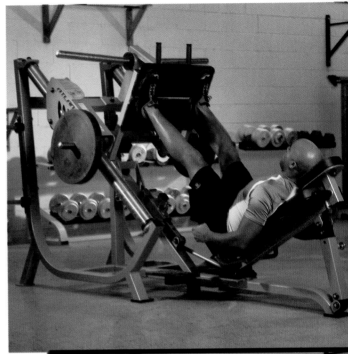

MUSCLE GROUP: quads and hamstrings

SETUP:

Adjust the pad on a leg-press machine to a forty-five-degree angle.

Lie on the pad and place your feet on the platform, slightly wider than your shoulders.

Push the weight slightly up and release the catch. Let the weight bend your legs until your knees are almost pressing into your chest.

STEP ONE: Push your feet against the platform as hard as possible, straightening your legs.

STEP TWO: Lower the weight again.

When you have completed your set, push the weight up again and lock the weight with the catch.

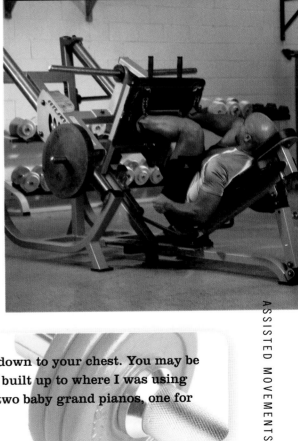

Tiki Tip: Make sure your knees come all the way down to your chest. You may be surprised by how much your thighs can handle. I built up to where I was using 1,100 pounds for 3 repetitions. That's like lifting two baby grand pianos, one for each quad.

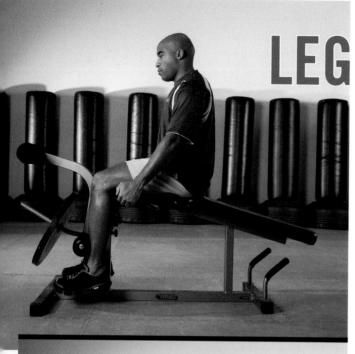

LEG EXTENSION

MUSCLE GROUP: quads

SETUP:

Sit in a leg-extension machine with the pads over the tops of your ankles.

Make sure your upper calves are roughly half an inch from the seat pad, and your knees are even with the machine's pivoting cam.

STEP ONE: Extend your legs (straightening them), and squeeze at the top of the movement.

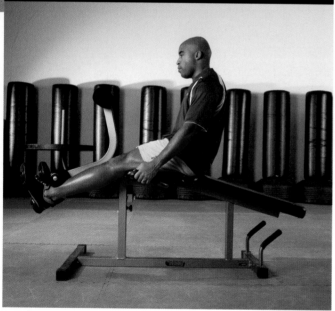

STEP TWO: Bring the weight back down, and do not allow your knees to go past ninety-degrees. This will help minimize knee stress. This particular exercise should be slow and deliberate.

Tiki Tip: There are a few different versions of this machine, but they all work the same way. Be careful to avoid jerky movements with this exercise. Using explosive force or momentum is a great way to tear up a knee.

LEG CURL

MUSCLE GROUP: hamstrings

SETUP:

Lie facedown on a leg-curl machine, chest flat on the bench. The back of your ankles should be against the pads, and your knees should be in line with the machine's rotating cam.

Grip the handgrips with both hands.

STEP ONE: Curl the weight with only the strength of the hamstrings.

STEP TWO: Squeeze at the top of the movement, and lower slowly back down.

Tiki Tip: Do not use momentum to swing the weight up and down, and do not allow your hips to come up off the bench during the movement. There is another variety of this machine where you sit straight up and push your legs down. The idea is the same: Focus on the backs of your legs, and don't use momentum.

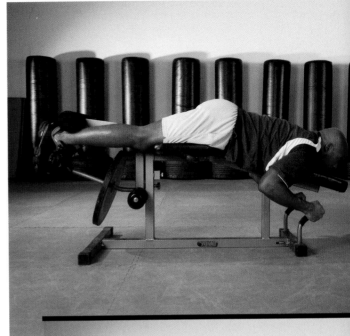

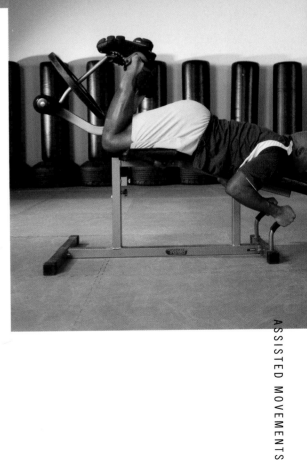

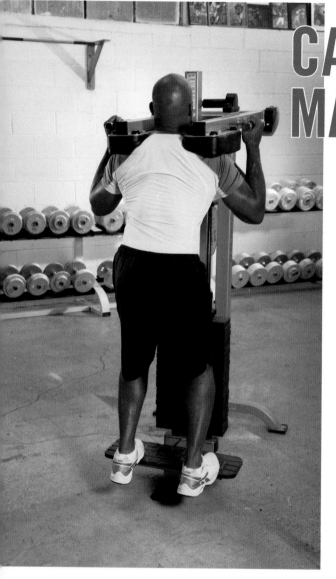

CALF RAISE MACHINE

MUSCLE GROUP: calves

SETUP:

Place your shoulders under the pads of the yoke with your back straight and place your toes and the balls of your feet on the toe block.

Push the weight up slightly, release the catch, and let the weight push you down so your heels are below your toes.

STEP ONE: Rise up as high as you can on your toes.

STEP TWO: Slowly return to the starting position.

Tiki Tip: To stretch your muscles correctly be sure to rise up as high as possible on your toes as you perform every repetition. Try varying the direction your toes point so you can work the muscle from all angles.

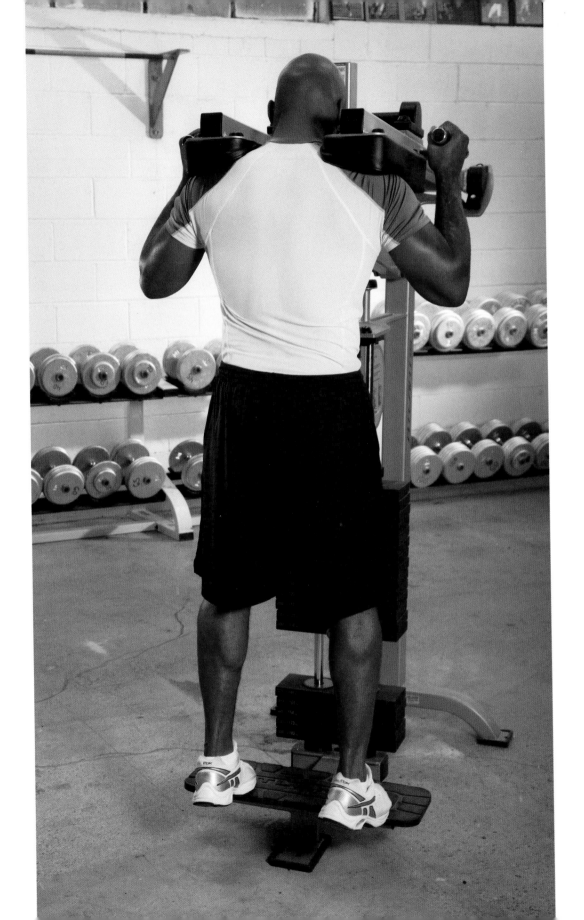

WRIST ROLLER

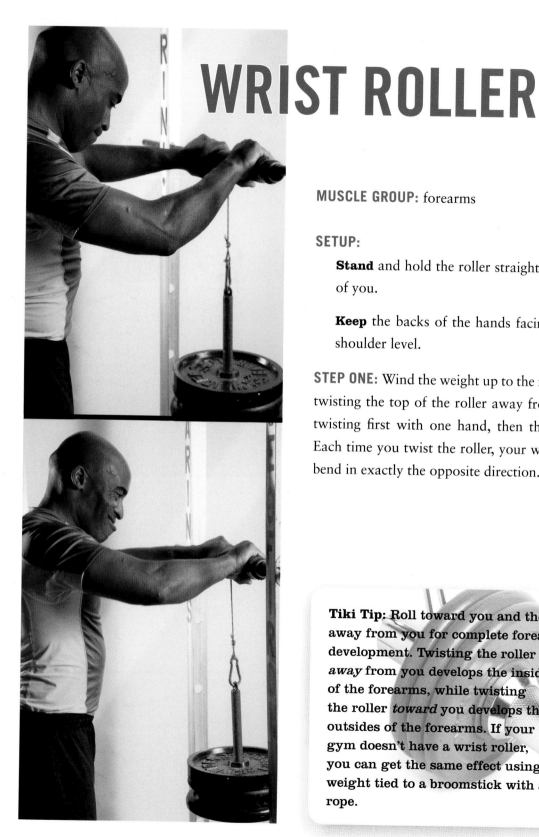

MUSCLE GROUP: forearms

SETUP:

> **Stand** and hold the roller straight in front of you.

> **Keep** the backs of the hands facing up at shoulder level.

STEP ONE: Wind the weight up to the roller by twisting the top of the roller away from you, twisting first with one hand, then the other. Each time you twist the roller, your wrist will bend in exactly the opposite direction.

Tiki Tip: Roll toward you and then away from you for complete forearm development. Twisting the roller *away* from you develops the insides of the forearms, while twisting the roller *toward* you develops the outsides of the forearms. If your gym doesn't have a wrist roller, you can get the same effect using a weight tied to a broomstick with a rope.

PLATE-LOADED GRIP

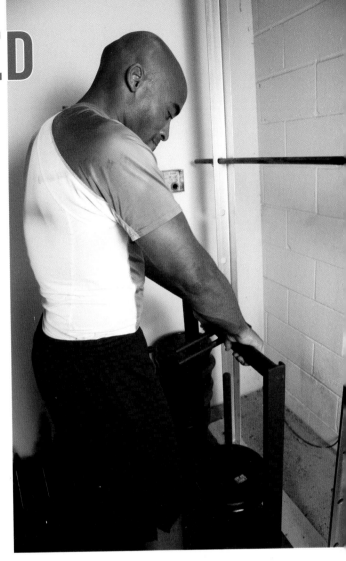

MUSCLE GROUP: fingers, wrists, and forearms

SETUP:

Load the plates, using whatever weight level your strength will allow.

STEP ONE: Standing or sitting, grab the two handles and squeeze your hands together so the handles of the plate-loaded machine touch.

Tiki Tip: You can work up to big poundage on a heavy-duty two-handed version. High reps or low reps both work the fingers and forearms to the max. Awesome movement for crushing power.

CHAPTER 10
ABDOMINALS/ CORE

The muscles in your midsection have numerous duties. They control the bending and twisting movements of your trunk, contribute to correct body posture, and form a protective external wall and internal support for your abdominal organs. It's no surprise, then, that working your abs will give you other benefits besides a flat stomach.

Ab workouts help prevent hernias and ruptures. They're important in enhancing your overall body strength, too. It never pays to ignore your abs.

The muscles of the front side of the abdomen are arranged in three layers. The fibers in each layer run in different directions similar to the layers of wood in a sheet of plywood. The result is a strong "girdle" of muscle that cov-ers and supports the abdominal cavity and the internal organs. The front of your abdomen gets the best workout from Crunches with feet elevated, Sit-ups with knees bent, and Incline Sit-ups.

Obliques are the strong muscles on either side of your waist that help you bend and twist. Usually, people who aren't in shape have weak stomach muscles and even weaker obliques. An athlete must train his obliques with the same intensity as he does other abdominal muscles. The obliques help stabilize the lower back while doing overhead lifting, squatting, picking a weight off the floor, or running. They are essential to a strong core.

Specifically, the external and internal oblique abdominal muscles, the ones at the sides of your waist, help you flex your entire trunk. Thus, they're partially developed by all types of Sit-up exercises. Besides contributing to flexibility, these muscles come into play with other important trunk movements, particularly those that involve your spine. You use them to flex your spine laterally—as when you bend from the hips and rotate your upper body.

Training your entire front area also helps you develop a strong, well-conditioned trunk and lower-back muscles. You must train your core using a combination of low and high repetitions to work both strength and endurance. High-repetition work can be done almost daily, provided the exercises are rotated. Lower-repetition work should be limited to two to three times per week to allow for the best recovery.

Here are the exercises you'll need for a complete abdominal workout.

SIT-UP

Lie on your back with your legs bent and your feet on the floor. Place your hands behind your neck or across your chest. Inhale and curl your torso off the floor. Exhale as you complete the movement. Return to the starting position without resting your torso on the floor.

SIT-UP

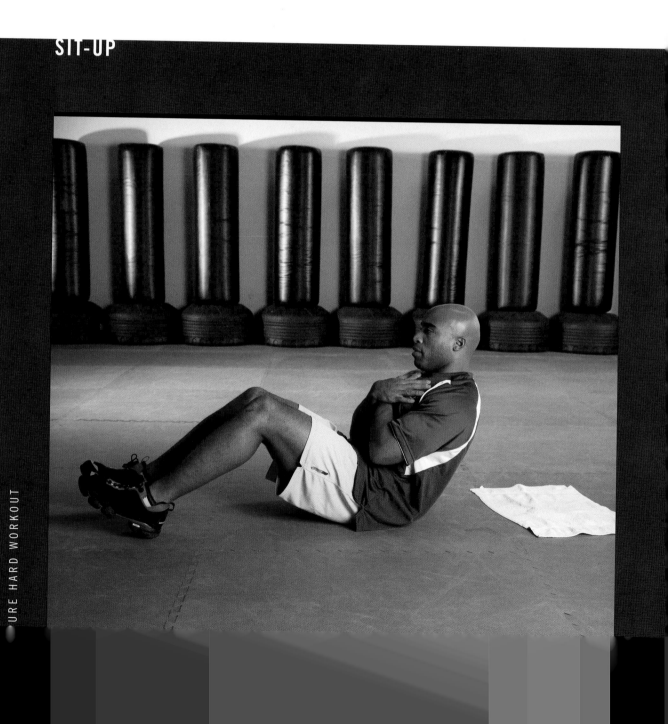

LYING LEG RAISE

Lie on your back with your hands behind your head. Raise your legs until they are straight up in the air, then lower them to the point just before they touch the ground. If this is too difficult, keep your knees bent during the motion and let your feet touch the ground at the bottom. When this gets too easy, have a partner restrict your legs with rubber bands.

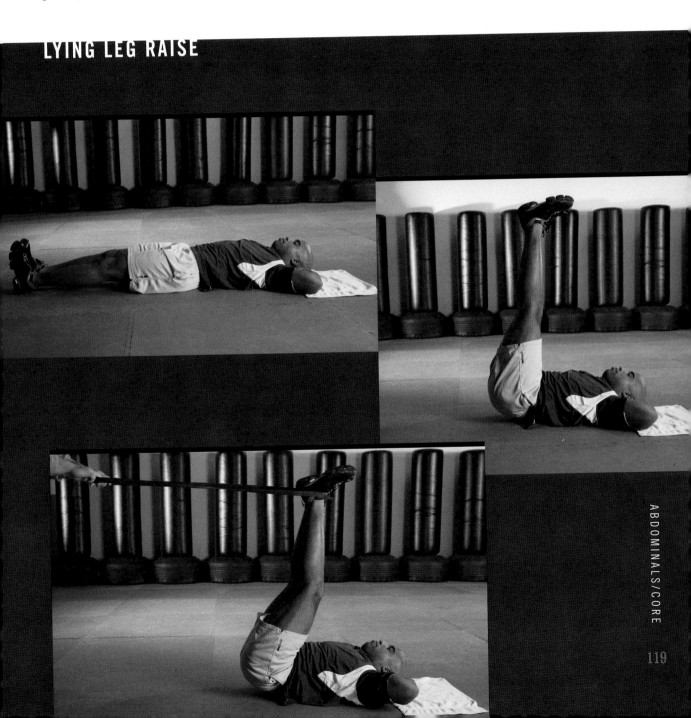

LYING LEG RAISE

ABDOMINALS/CORE

HANGING LEG RAISE

Hang from a pull bar and bring your legs up and in front of you at a ninety-degree angle. Avoid swinging. You can either hang straight from the bar or use supports around your upper arms, as Tiki does. An easier version involves bending your legs and bringing up your knees. You can also do Leg and Knee Raises on a Dip stand. Support yourself with elbows locked.

HANGING LEG RAISE

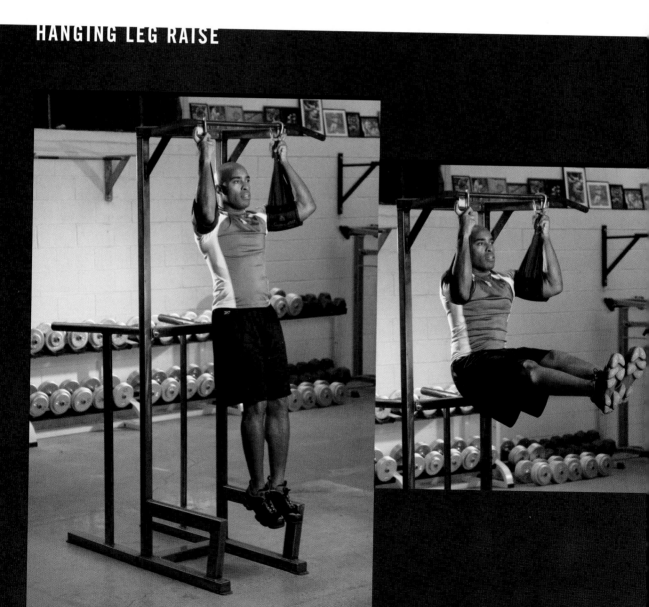

KNEE LIFT ON A DIP STAND

DECLINE SIT-UP

Rest your elbows on the support pads and position the lumbar support pad in the small part of your back. Inhale and pull your knees up to your chest, rounding your back to contract your abdominals correctly. Exhale as you complete the movement.

Lie on a decline bench and hook your feet under the roller pads. Place your hands behind your head. Pull your torso up, using your abs and exhaling as you complete the movement. As you get better at this, incorporate a twist to the side as you rise, as Tiki does. This stresses the abs even more.

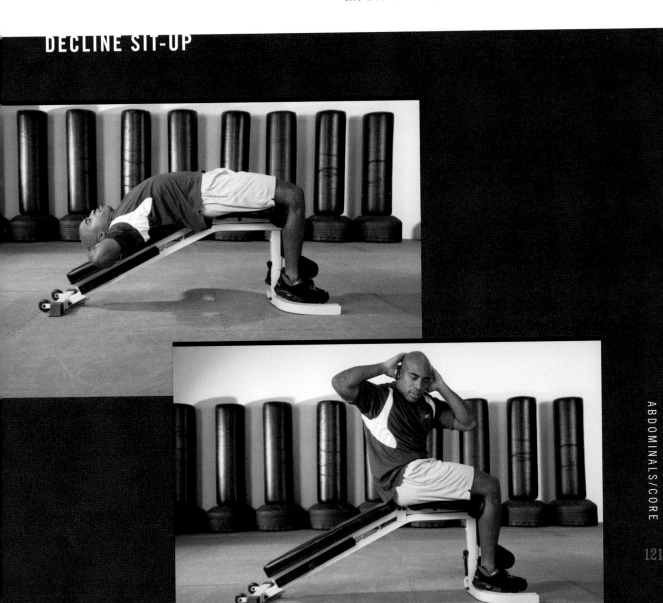

DECLINE SIT-UP

ABDOMINALS/CORE

121

MEDICINE BALL WORK

Pass the ball to a training partner or use a medicine ball rebounder. Mini trampoline passes work the entire upper body, particularly the shoulder girdle and trunk. High repetitions or even a light weight will tax your cardiovascular system.

MEDICINE BALL WORK

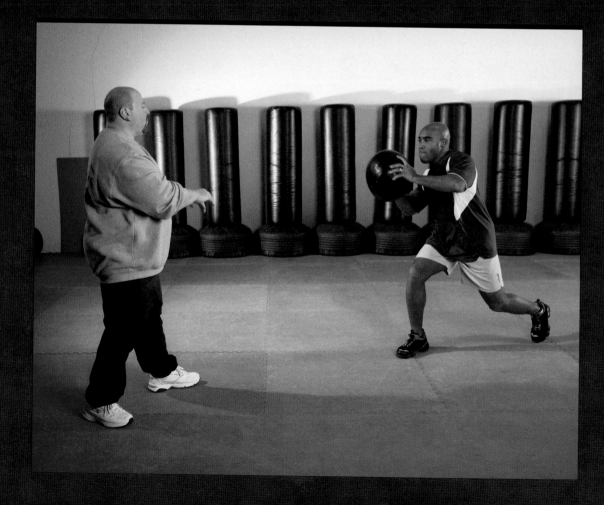

RUSSIAN TWIST

Sit on the floor in a half sit-up position with your feet anchored under a bench. Hold a medicine ball, dumbbell, or weight at arm's length from your chest. Twist side to side, using the power of your trunk. You can also do this in a standing position. A common mistake is to move the weight using only your arms. Be sure to do this motion using abdominals only.

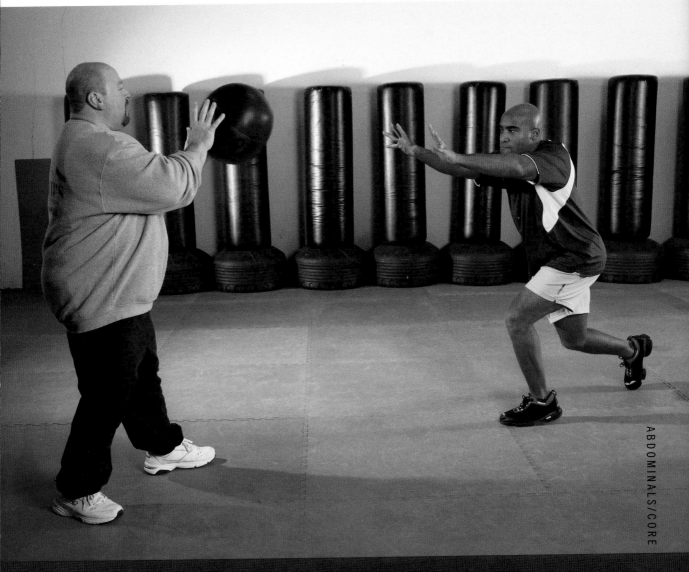

CABLE CRUNCH

Kneel down in front of a weight stack and grab a triceps rope roughly even with your head. Crunch down, rounding your back and pulling down on the rope. Exhale as you do so.

CABLE CRUNCH

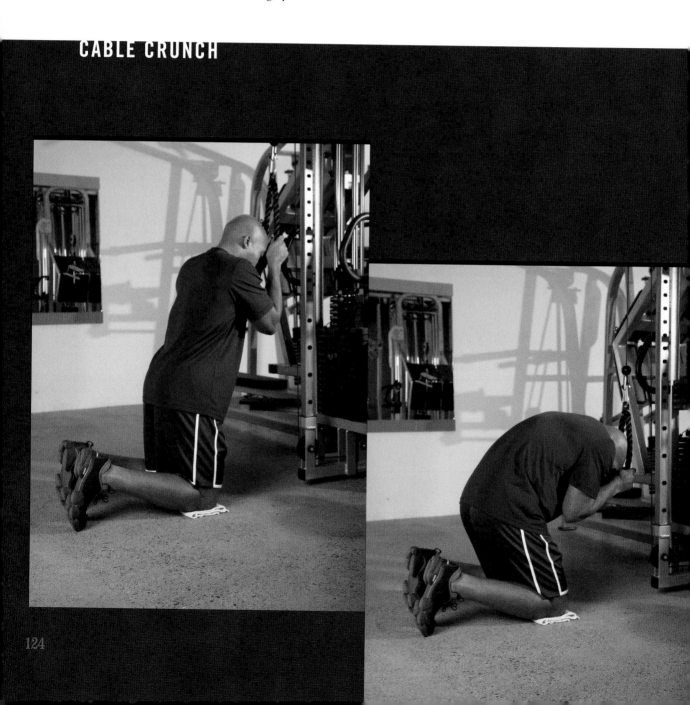

DUMBBELL
SIDE BEND

Stand with your feet slightly apart, holding the dumbbell in your right hand. Bend your torso to the right side as far as you can.

Return to the starting position. After a set, switch hands and bend to the opposite side.

DUMBBELL SIDE BEND

ABDOMINALS/CORE

125

WINDMILL

Stand up straight with both hands overhead. Bend forward, twisting your body as you descend until you touch the floor with your hands. Reverse the motion and return to the start position. As you get better at this, hold a weight or a medicine ball in your hands. The arms remain straight throughout the exercise even when holding the weights. Look up at the weight as you do each rep and keep it directly over your body. Windmills are difficult at first, even with modest weight—use only weight you can control.

WINDMILL

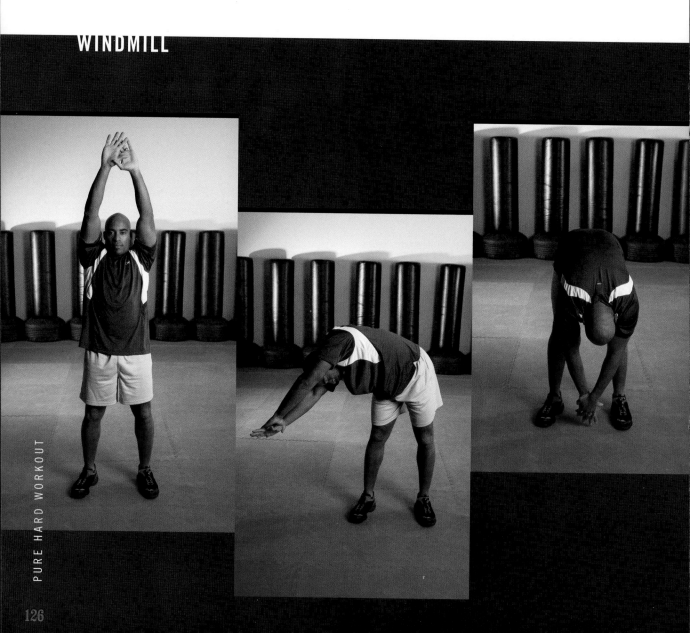

BICYCLE CRUNCH

Lie on your back with your hands behind your head. Bring your left knee toward your head as you crunch up and touch it with your right elbow. Straighten your leg and relax your upper body. Next, bring your right knee and left elbow together. Make sure the opposite leg is fully extended.

BICYCLE CRUNCH

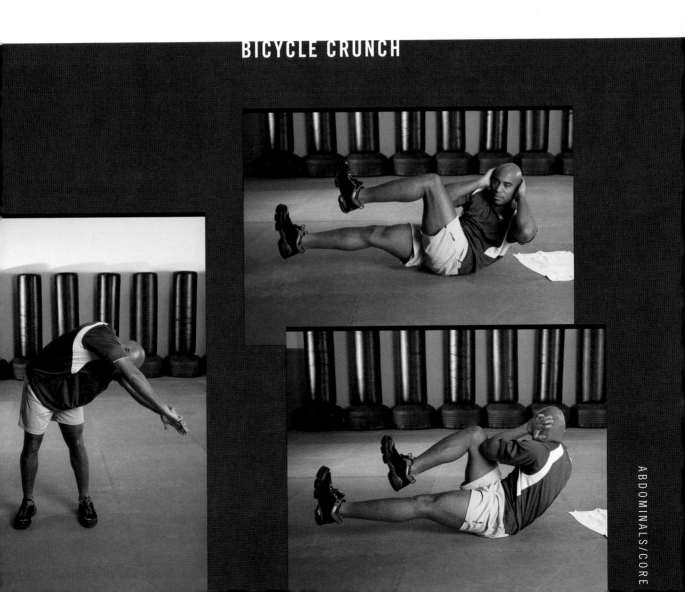

WOOD CHOPPER

Hold a weight in one or both hands. Starting high on one side, bring the weight down to the low position on the other side as if you were using an ax. Swing the weight by using the power of your trunk rather than the arms. Pivot on the balls of your feet.

KNEE KICK/ MOUNTAIN CLIMBER

Get into a push-up position with one leg extended and the other pulled in toward your chest. In one motion, bring your extended leg into your chest and extend your tucked leg so that you're in the same position on the opposite side.

PLANK HOLD

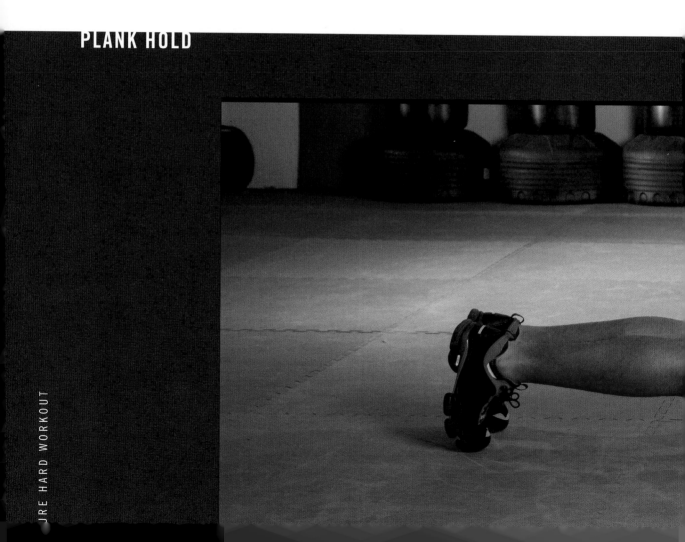

PLANK
HOLD

Lie on your stomach with your forearms underneath your chest. Raise up onto your forearms and your toes. You're basically in a push-up position, but your forearms are supporting your upper body instead of your hands. Keep your back straight and hold for as long as possible.

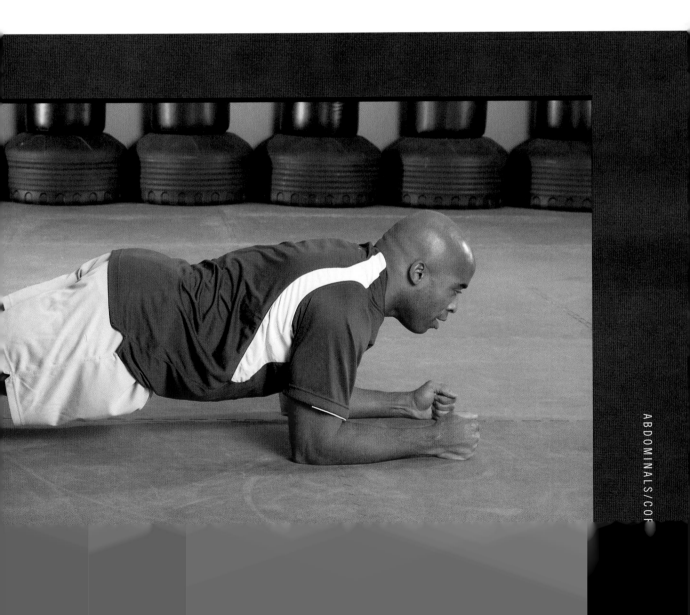

Every individual is unique, and his motivation to train is personal. We each possess our own levels of natural and learned abilities. Each of us must recognize our own proficiency level and set priorities accordingly. If you set a goal to become stronger, it must be your highest priority, and you must be willing to make the necessary sacrifices to reach your goal.

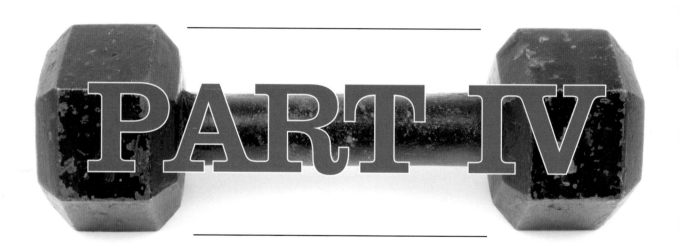

PART IV

The journey is a long hard road, but with each workout you'll see and feel the rewards. You'll see yourself growing, and you'll gain confidence and discover that you're better able to handle many challenges in life. The committed athlete will return to his workouts as a source of inner strength. When you build a →

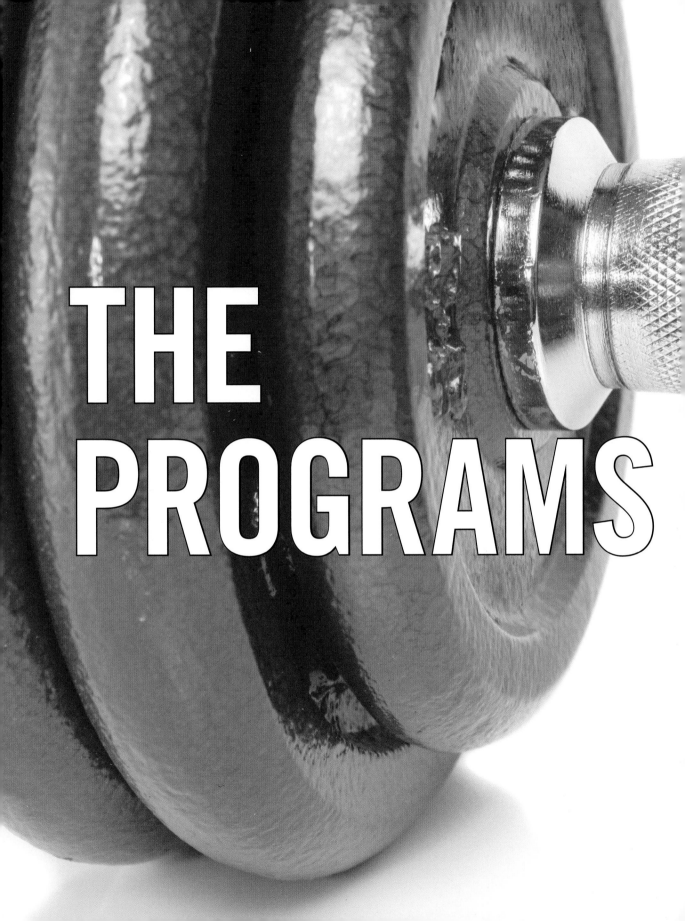

THE PROGRAMS

house one brick at a time, the foundation eventually becomes strong enough to hold the weight of the entire building. So, too, will your training, one workout at a time, build a body that's capable of sustained physical effort.

Regardless of the inevitable setbacks, personal distractions, and even injuries if they happen, you must keep focused and find a way to meet your goal. If a person wants it badly enough, he'll find a way to reach it. He'll squeeze in a workout during a busy day, or find the motivation to head to the gym when he thinks he's too tired. Personal choices will determine how far a person will go with his training. Make no mistake about the effort required: It will take a burning desire and prolonged steady effort.

At times, your desire will be intense and the work physically demanding but satisfying. At other times your desire will be there, but the motivation to work will be missing. Regardless of the balance, you must give your best effort to each and every workout, week after week, month after month, year after year. Don't be discouraged. Don't dwell on negative thoughts, and stay away from negative people who have nothing positive to contribute to your life.

Gradually learn how to train hard and heavy; pure hard work doesn't mean using a light set of weights and doing a lot of reps to get a pump. It means using the heaviest possible weight for the most reps you can manage while maintaining good execution of the movement. Never be satisfied with what you've been doing.

Sure, it's important to stop long enough to reward yourself when you reach a goal—enjoy a good meal or take a night off—but always strive to go beyond your limits and push yourself to new heights. You must develop mental toughness as you build physical strength.

Remember that tough times don't last, but tough people do. Also, don't use age as a stumbling block. It shouldn't be a factor. I had my best season at an age considered old for an NFL running back. I never approached my training as an "old" player, simply because Joe would never allow that to be an excuse. Neither should anyone who's serious about training hard. If you follow the program in this book, you'll get the best results in the least amount of time—even though you'll have to grit your teeth in the process.

—TIKI

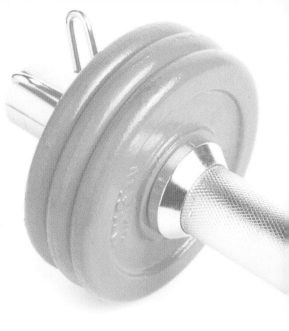

CHAPTER 11
ASSESSING AND MEASURING

The basic measurement for classifying beginner, intermediate, and advanced athletes is the amount of work they can recuperate from. Time is part of this equation because it takes longer to recuperate as you lift heavier weights. A beginner will not have nearly the endurance or recuperation ability of an advanced athlete.

The training approaches for each of these three fitness levels are vastly different from the others. The beginner's workout must be short, and the intensity level has to be kept down. This will ensure that his overall health isn't overburdened.

A beginner should train three times per week. A person of average health who wants to improve physically should stick to this schedule for the first year. The increase in his muscle size and strength should dictate future training goals. Someone with natural athletic abilities

ONE-REP MAXIMUM

One-rep max is the maximum amount of weight you can heft once for a particular lift. Nobody can lift 100 percent of their strength during every workout, so you have to break this down into percentages. Once you establish your current one-rep max, then dial back to a productive 70 to 85 percent of that amount. It's the best way to keep your progress going in a steady, positive way. Every three to four weeks, determine a new 100 percent maximum and begin all over again. You'll be building strength every step of the way.

and in excellent physical condition can gradually increase the intensity of his training. Time will dictate when to turn up the intensity. A beginner just wants to get through a workout. As he gets stronger, he'll be able to handle more weight and greater intensity.

Many beginners feel that if a little exercise is good, then a whole lot will be better. Nothing could be further from the truth. A person has only so much training energy to spare. Using any more than you're capable of giving won't help you gain muscle or strength any faster. And rest time is just as important to muscle growth as lifting is.

When a person feels ready to up the level of his workout, he should experiment with the intermediate routine—for example, substituting one intermediate workout for one of his beginner workouts and seeing how he feels. This will help him determine if he's ready. A beginner can use much of the material in this book when he reaches the intermediate stage of his physical and strength development. The same formulas, tips, and cautions apply, and most of the exercises are the same except for increasing the amount of weight used. An intermediate person should train four to five times per week.

Ultimately, transitioning from the intermediate level to the advanced level will depend on how long you've been training, how hard you've been training, and if you feel ready to go harder and longer. More difficult exercise schedules will provide more intensity. The exercises basically remain the same but become more challenging by adding either extra sets or more weight, or both.

VOLUME AND INTENSITY

You must calculate how much useful gross work in the medium- to high-intensity stuff you're performing during your regular workouts. The volume of work will eventually enable you to gain in physical strength—due to the intensity load—and also gain in overall development and cardiovascular efficiency.

When determining what constitutes "valuable volume" in your training, you must figure out what percentile you use for most of your sets and repetitions. In other words, you first want to determine what your maximum is and how much of your workout will be done at that level. The guidelines in this book will help you determine just what volume of work will help you the most, and the point at which effort results in physical depletion without a corresponding increase in muscle mass or strength.

Volume refers to the amount of weight you lift (sets multiplied by reps multiplied by weight). Every athlete needs to know how much is too much. Never overtrain. It's counterproductive. You can gauge it by the rate at which you recover from workout to workout. When your workouts grow longer and longer, but your maximum performance in repetitions and poundage remain the same, then it's safe to say that most of the added work is done in vain. This would mean that you might have chosen too light a weight for the desired repetitions, or else the repetition scheme was too low for the amount of resistance. In either situation, you're wasting your valuable training time and doing little or nothing for your strength.

The most functional weight to be used for the majority of your training time should be between 75 percent and 80 percent of your maximum poundage. For example, if you can bench-press 315 pounds, your most efficient weight for sets and repetitions would be

about 255 pounds. You could use the double- and/or triple-progression method (or pyramid system), increasing the weight, the reps, and/or the sets at the same time. Powerlifters have used variations of this method for years. Or you could use the heavy-singles method (one rep at near-maximum weight). It all depends on what you're attempting to achieve.

Beginning trainees should remember that much of the material in this book can be used when they reach the intermediate and advanced stages of their physical development. Until then, focus on the proper forms for each exercise in this book.

ASSESSING YOUR WORKOUTS

Each workout will build strength, muscular endurance, and confidence. The progress you achieve week to week will be built incrementally with each lift. Sometimes you will progress by just 1 more pound on the bar; sometimes you'll have strength breakthroughs.

It's all about perseverance. Some people begin by telling themselves they're going to work out so many times a week, and they do this with all the enthusiasm they can muster. Eventually, though, their interest wanes, usually because they've set too unrealistic a goal, and they don't have the heart to follow through with the plan. So they fail the program, and fail themselves. All this accomplishes is to make them less willing to try again.

THE NINE FACES OF STRENGTH

Here are nine classifications of strength. It's always important to know what you're doing and why. You can measure your eccentric strength or speed strength or speed endurance by understanding each of these nine faces of strength.

1. **Concentric strength**: Your one-rep maximum in a movement.
2. **Eccentric strength**: Your one-rep maximum while lowering a weight under control. (Add 40 percent to your concentric strength.)
3. **Static strength**: Your maximum holding strength in a given position. (Add 2 percent to your concentric strength.)
4. **Limit strength**: The same as concentric strength except you're under the influence of muscle-building drugs, hypnosis, or other techniques that elevate your potential for strength output beyond what it would normally be.
5. **Speed strength**: Starting strength; your ability to recruit a maximum number of muscle fibers simultaneously.
6. **Explosive strength**: Your ability to keep the fibers firing over time.
7. **Anaerobic power**: Local muscle endurance; your ability to continue submaximal force output over a long period.
8. **Strength endurance**: Your ability to put forth maximum muscular contractures time after time with no appreciable decline in force output.
9. **Speed endurance**: Your ability to maintain your maximum speed over distance.

Strength training requires improving your strength levels while decreasing your transition time (i.e., eccentric to concentric). You must also increase your starting force, your max force, your transition max force, and your explosive strength.

Eventually it will seem impossible to add weight to the bar on a regular basis. You must keep training at your top poundage over and over for long periods of time. Always work as hard as you possibly can. Eventually, your efforts will make you even stronger.

Successful weight training takes tenacity and patience. Start by setting short-term goals from workout to workout. Strive to lift more in a Squat, Bench Press, Deadlift, or other exercise, and you'll progress. It's important to add weight to the bar every time you lift. That's how you'll coax those muscles and your body to grow. The more weight you can handle in the exercises you do, the stronger and thicker your tendons, ligaments, and muscles will get. That's the key to creating real body strength.

Joe's training with Tiki emphasized this technique. Tiki's body weight increased from 183 pounds to 208 pounds, and he ended up with three times more strength and endurance. This was accomplished through hard, heavy workouts that were progressively more grueling. Without adding weights to the bar, you won't see results, and consequently, you won't be motivated to put in the hard work.

It's easy to become frustrated and lose interest if you're working hard but not getting any stronger. That's the case for people who follow the same routine without challenging their muscles. The great thing about weight training is that you *can* challenge your muscles incrementally, by adding a 1- or 2-pound plate to the bar. Even if you stick with the same exercises and reps, you'll see a difference. And those pounds eventually add up to 5- or 10-pound plates. Then you'll really start seeing results.

Some people weigh themselves every day to see if they've gained weight, but they don't take into account whether it's usable muscle weight. Usable weight gain means being able to lift the barbell more easily because you've built some solid muscle. If you're putting on weight but still struggling with your workout, you're probably taking in more calories than you're burning, meaning that you're adding fat, not muscle.

Others assess their progress by taking body measurements with a tape measure to see if they've gained 1 or 2 inches here and there.

Some men like to measure their arms and chests to see if they've gained mass in those areas. Bodybuilders especially like to use the tape. But serious weightlifters don't regard a scale or a tape measure as a helpful means of assessing their gains. Instead, you should judge your progress by how much weight you're able to move.

A note on rest time: The amount of rest time you take between sets depends on what exercise you're doing. For instance, if you're in good condition and can move fairly quickly with the heavy Squats and Deadlifts (and some people go at them in 1 to 2 minutes), then you can rest, say, 2 minutes or so, depending on how heavy the set. The 4-, 5-, and 6-hour weekly programs are designed to add more exercises as well as a set or two to the core lifts, so your rest periods should increase in proportion to the effort you're putting out. If you're as focused and motivated about the workout as you should be, then you should never lag or waste time with distractions. You're going to see a lot of exercises to get done in these programs, but keep in mind that Tiki got through these programs in 90 minutes or less. If it's taking you longer than that, you're lagging.

You'll learn to recognize a signal that goes off in your brain telling you to go lift some weight. Learn to pay attention to this as well as the pace of your workouts. If you're too slow, you won't accomplish enough work during your allotted time to force your body to grow stronger.

SIX GOALS WORTH ACHIEVING

As we've repeatedly emphasized throughout this book, you're taking on a tremendous challenge in following this program. You'll need patience, discipline, and single-minded determination to succeed. To help you find your focus, consider the following six recommendations as tools to be used alongside the weights. You can apply them to your short-term goals, and keep them in mind during the long haul. They'll help you stay motivated and on track.

1. Make your training a challenge. Get into it. Set a commitment goal and stick to it.
2. Construct and reconstruct your workouts, but don't overanalyze them. As your knowledge and experience grow, you'll devise more ways to avoid getting bored and get the most out of your training.
3. Establish a workout plan and avoid interrupting influences. Quit wasting your time talking with people who aren't training properly. Get to know yourself. Learn what motivates you.
4. Get aggressive in the gym; become one of the strongest guys in there. Your program should be your sole focus. You don't have time to let weak individuals distract you or bring you down.
5. Judge yourself by how much stronger and bigger you're becoming. Heavy training will remake you, and your mental and emotional health will improve in direct proportion.
6. Have faith in yourself and believe you can become strong. Once you become hooked on working out consistently, perseverance and tenacity become a way of life. Let the pure hard work outlined in this book inspire and transform you.

CHAPTER 12
BEGINNER PROGRAM

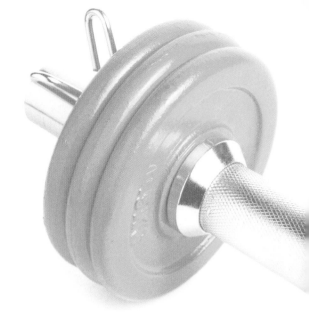

So you want to work out. You've made up your mind that you're willing to invest the effort and time it will take. You hope you'll be disciplined enough to follow through. Keep in mind that most people you meet in a gym aren't training properly and have no idea what real training is all about.

Don't confuse bodybuilding with strength training. The first involves building cosmetic muscle; strength training will be slower and harder, but it will give

you more solid results in the end. Work at your own pace and don't add more weights to the bar or move on to the next level until you feel confident in your progress. If you are not sure, experiment. Add a small amount of weight for one exercise and see how it feels.

Follow the steps outlined in this book and your quest toward excellence will succeed.

Step one for the beginner means developing a solid foundation. These instructions describe exactly what exercises to do, how often to do them, and the amount of weight to use. A *repetition* (rep) is one movement with the barbell or weight machine. A *set* is a group of repetitions.

There is a science to determining the proper number of reps and sets you'll need to do. High reps with light weights produce muscle changes that will build endurance. Lower reps with heavier weights produce stronger muscles, which is the goal we all seek. When your muscles are too fatigued to do another set at a high level of intensity, then you've done the right number of sets.

Normally, you should be able to do 3 to 5 sets if you put the proper amount of intensity into the exercise. When lifting your maximum percentage of weight, you should rest 3 to 5 minutes between sets to allow your muscles time to recover and get your heart rate down to a normal level. The time it takes your muscles to recuperate between workouts varies from one individual to another, but you should aim to work out three days a week to start.

During the first few weeks of following the program in *Tiki Barber's Pure Hard Workout*, you should work into your routine slowly. Don't rush your progress. Be honest with yourself about how much weight you can—or can't—handle, and take the time to learn to do the movement perfectly. It won't be long before you'll be able to perform at a maximum level.

When a beginner starts a strength or bodybuilding program, he often believes he should be working out every day. This won't help you reach your goals at a faster rate. More often, pushing yourself inappropriately will hamper your ability to adjust mentally to the regimen. It can also increase the risk of injury. If by training too fast you tear muscles or experience severe soreness, this will certainly deter your motivation. You'll enjoy your workouts more when you experience the hard work in a healthy frame of mind and body.

Older people will recover at a slower rate, as will people with larger muscles. Heavy training for strength takes a longer recuperation period than lighter training for endurance. The better your overall fitness level, the shorter the recuperation time will be between workouts. That's why in the beginning, the average person should work out three times per week.

For most people, Mondays, Wednesdays, and Fridays work best, but tailor it to your schedule. The beginning of training requires the hardest work and the most effort. The rest between workouts will be longer. We can't emphasize enough how important it is to recuperate fully before another hard training session. As time goes by and your experience grows, you'll reach a point where hard training won't be so totally fatiguing. It is at this point that you'll be able to better embrace the advanced training program. You'll also need to increase your discipline because it's easy to start backsliding when you reach this level.

Another critical mistake a beginner can make is to avoid the more difficult exercises such as Squats, Bent-Over Rows, heavy Bench Presses, or Deadlifts. For instance, Leg Extensions or Hack Squats won't replace the power and benefit you'll get from heavy Squats. Rest assured that the Pure Hard Workout program will have you hitting the *real* exercises.

If your goal is to become a stronger, better athlete, you need muscle weight. You should dedicate your training time and energy toward this goal. Many people who are new at training will often waste time and energy performing half-decent exercises in place of the correct movements. They're tempted to do them because those exercises are easier to perform and require less effort. Light weights won't build true power, nor will they build useful bulk. In order to gain bulk and power, you can't continually drain your energy by doing unproductive exercises. As discussed early in the nutrition chapter, don't neglect to increase your caloric intake as you get bigger and stronger.

Learn to adjust your workout so that it fits into your allotted time schedule. Every workout should be followed through to the end, and then varied if you become burned out from too many sets or reps of a particular exercise. You can add or subtract an exercise from time to time, but the basic routine will pack on muscle and functional strength throughout your body, which is the most important goal.

DAY ONE (legs and chest)

WARM-UP: Stretch for 5 minutes, especially the lower lumbar muscles and hamstrings. Do Hyperextensions, 2 sets of 10 reps.

- Leg Press (page 109)
- Calf Raise Machine (pages 112–13)
- Squat (pages 54–55)
- Bench Press (pages 56–57)
- Incline Bench Press (page 66)
- Decline Bench Press (page 67)
- Dip (page 77)
- Dumbbell Fly (page 71)
- Dumbbell Pullover (page 72)

LEG PRESS

3 sets of 10 reps using 50 percent of your body weight

CALF PRESS

3 sets of 8 to 10 reps using 50 percent of your body weight

SQUAT

1 set of 10 reps using 40 percent of your body weight, then do 3 sets of 6 reps using 65 percent of your body weight

BENCH PRESS

1 set of 10 reps with 50 percent of maximum weight, then 4 sets of 6 reps with 65 percent of maximum bench-press weight

INCLINE BENCH PRESS

3 sets of 8 reps with 55 percent of maximum bench-press weight

DECLINE BENCH PRESS

3 sets of 8 to 10 reps with 55 percent of maximum bench-press weight

DIP

3 sets of 5 to 7 reps of your body weight (if they're too difficult, there are machines that can assist; if no machine is available, start with 10 to 25 Push-ups per set until you build up your repetitions)

DUMBBELL FLY

3 sets of 8 to 10 reps using light dumbbells

DUMBBELL PULLOVER

3 sets of 12 to 15 reps using light dumbbells

DAY TWO (shoulders and arms)

WARM-UP: Stretch for 5 minutes. Do Hyper-extensions, 2 sets of 10 reps.

- Seated Press (page 69)
- Military Press (page 58)
- Lateral Raise (page 79)
- Upright Row (page 80)
- Shrug (page 81)
- Triceps Pushdown (page 105)
- Standing Triceps Extension (page 89)
- Standing Barbell Curl (page 83)
- Dumbbell Hammer Curl (page 95)
- Seated Wrist Curl (page 97)

SEATED PRESS

4 sets of 6 to 8 reps using 55 percent of maximum bench-press weight

MILITARY PRESS

4 sets of 6 to 8 reps with medium-weight dumbbells

LATERAL RAISE

3 sets of 8 reps with medium weight

UPRIGHT ROW

3 sets of 8 to 10 reps using medium weight

SHRUG

4 sets of 8 to 10 reps with heavy weight

TRICEPS PUSHDOWN

3 sets of 8 to 10 reps using heavy weight on a cable

STANDING TRICEPS EXTENSION

3 sets of 8 to 10 reps using heavy weight, standing or seated

STANDING BARBELL CURL

3 sets of 6 to 8 reps using medium weight

DUMBBELL HAMMER CURL

3 sets of 8 to 10 reps with medium weight

SEATED WRIST CURL

4 sets of 10 to 12 reps

DAY THREE (back and abdominals)

WARM-UP: Stretch for 5 minutes. Do Hyper-extensions, 2 sets of 10 reps.

- Lat Pulldown (page 100)
- T-Bar Row (page 104)
- Bent-Over Row (page 74)
- Deadlift (pages 59–61)
- Dumbbell One-Arm Row (page 73)
- Cable Row (page 103)
- Sit-up (page 118)
- Lying Leg Raise (page 119)
- Dumbbell Side Bend (page 125)

LAT PULLDOWN

3 sets of 10 reps with medium weight

T-BAR ROW

3 sets of 8 reps with medium weight

BENT-OVER ROW

3 sets of 8 reps using medium weight

DEADLIFT

4 sets of 6 reps with medium weight

DUMBBELL ONE-ARM ROW

3 sets of 10 reps with heavy dumbbells

CABLE ROW

3 sets of 8 reps with medium weight

SIT-UP

3 sets of 10 to 15 reps (if this exercise becomes too easy, place a 10-pound plate on your chest or do them on a decline bench)

LYING LEG RAISE

3 sets of 10 to 15 reps (if this exercise becomes too easy, put on ankle weights or squeeze a dumbbell between your feet for added resistance; a medicine ball can also be used)

DUMBBELL SIDE BEND

3 sets of 15 reps (use a medium to heavy dumbbell)

CHAPTER 13
INTERMEDIATE PROGRAM

The training time for the intermediate program increases at a much faster rate than that for the beginner. For openers, the heavier weights that have become necessary require more warm-up sets than are necessary for the beginner stage. This will mean adding to the volume of work over time. You must also realize that at the intermediate level, the intensity of your workouts has increased. The challenge here is figuring out how to do more work, which is also harder work, without becoming stale or discouraged.

At this time a split routine (dividing your schedule so that muscle groups have time to recuperate between workouts) must be incorporated into your training. You'll want to divide up your workout routines so that you're training four times per week. At each session, the work will increase and the routine will become harder.

It's also necessary at this time to distribute the workload of the various lifts and exercises.

The goal is to develop a more sophisticated method of handling the training load and intensity without getting burned out or injured. This is more complicated than it sounds. It becomes harder to develop strength when you're already fairly strong. This is because you're already functioning close to your maximum potential. From here on out, your gains will slow down, so it's important to take this into account and not become discouraged.

The intermediate routines outlined in this chapter will eliminate the guesswork or the need to experiment with other techniques and methods, which will claim energy that would be better used focusing on the more intense intermediate phase. They will also allow you to perform at your peak intensity while permitting your muscles to recuperate and grow.

You can measure your success by the routine. If you can't adapt to the increased workload, your workouts will suffer. Your energy will be depleted, and your strength level will decrease. So take it slowly and carefully. You must begin by developing the ability to recuperate from the stimulus of volume, which in time will create the ability to work for longer periods.

Rest assured, eventually you'll adapt to a heavy workload. Also, if you find the workout too long you can always finish the exercises on another day. Once you get your exercises and time between sets down, and if you don't spend your time talking and fooling around, you can definitely get through a workout in a reasonable time.

DAY ONE (legs and upper body)

WARM-UP: Stretch for 5 minutes. Do Hyper-extensions, 2 sets of 10 reps.

- Leg Press (page 109)
- Squat (pages 54–55)
- Good Morning (page 84)
- Calf Raise Machine (pages 112–13)
- Leg Extension (page 110)
- Leg Curl (page 111)
- Bench Press (pages 56–57)
- Incline Bench Press (page 66)
- Dip or Decline Bench Press (pages 67, 77)
- Dumbbell Fly (page 71)
- Dumbbell Pullover (page 72)

LEG PRESS

- 1 set of 10 reps at 50 percent of your body weight
- 2 sets of 8 reps at 70 percent of maximum leg-press weight
- 3 sets of 5 reps at 80 percent of maximum leg-press weight

SQUAT

- 1 set of 10 reps at 50 percent of maximum weight
- 1 set of 5 reps at 75 percent of maximum weight
- 4 sets of 3 reps at 85 percent of maximum weight

GOOD MORNING

3 sets of 8 reps at 50 percent of maximum Squat weight

CALF RAISE MACHINE

3 sets of 8 to 10 reps of heavy weight

LEG EXTENSION

3 sets of 8 to 10 reps at medium to heavy weight

LEG CURL

3 sets of 10 reps at medium weight

BENCH PRESS

- 1 set of 15 reps with just the bar
- 1 set of 10 reps at light weight
- 1 set of 5 reps at 70 percent of maximum weight
- 4 sets of 2 to 3 reps at 87 percent of maximum weight

INCLINE BENCH PRESS

3 to 4 sets of 5 to 7 reps at 70 percent of bench-press weight

DIP OR DECLINE BENCH PRESS

3 sets of 6 to 8 reps (when Dips become too easy with your own body weight, add resistance with either dumbbells or plates strapped around your waist)

DUMBBELL FLY

3 to 4 sets of 6 to 8 reps at medium to heavy dumbbell weight

DUMBBELL PULLOVER

2 to 3 sets of 10 to 12 reps

DAY TWO (shoulders, arms, and abdominals)

WARM-UP: Stretch for 5 minutes. Do Hyper-extensions, 2 sets of 10 reps.

- Military Press (page 58)
- Lateral Raise (page 79)
- Upright Row (page 80)
- Bent-Over Lateral (page 78)
- Shrug (page 81)
- Triceps Pushdown (page 105)
- Triceps Lying Extension (page 90)
- Close-Grip Bench Press (page 68)
- Standing Barbell Curl (page 88)
- Preacher Curl (page 94)
- Incline Dumbbell Curl (page 93)
- Sit-up (page 118)
- Russian Twist (page 123)
- Hanging Leg Raise (page 120)
- Seated Wrist Curl (page 97)

MILITARY PRESS

- 1 set of 15 reps with light weight (to get shoulders and triceps warmed up)
- 1 set of 10 reps using light weight
- 4 to 5 sets of 5 to 7 reps with medium to heavy weight

LATERAL RAISE

3 sets of 5 to 6 reps

UPRIGHT ROW

3 sets of 8 to 10 reps with medium weight (use barbells or dumbbells)

BENT-OVER LATERAL

3 sets of 8 to 10 reps using medium to heavy weight on dumbbells

SHRUG (BARBELL, DUMBBELLS, OR SHRUG MACHINE)

4 to 5 sets of 5 to 7 reps using heavy weights

TRICEPS PUSHDOWN

3 to 4 sets of 8 to 10 reps with heavy weight

TRICEPS LYING EXTENSION

3 to 4 sets of 6 to 8 reps at heavy weight

CLOSE-GRIP BENCH PRESS

3 to 4 sets of 6 reps using 60 to 65 percent of your maximum bench-press weight

STANDING BARBELL CURL

4 sets of 6 to 8 reps with heavy weight (just don't use weight that's so heavy that your form gets ugly)

PREACHER CURL

3 sets of 6 to 8 reps

INCLINE DUMBBELL CURL

SIT-UP

3 sets of 12 to 15 reps, add resistance when the reps get too easy

RUSSIAN TWIST

3 sets of 10 reps

HANGING LEG RAISE

3 sets of 15 to 20 reps at body weight

SEATED WRIST CURL

3 sets of 10 reps using heavy weight

DAY THREE (back)

- Lat Pulldown (page 100)
- T-Bar Row (page 104)
- Deadlift (pages 59–61)
- Bent-Over Row (page 74)
- Chin-up or Pull-up (pages 75 and 76)
- Hyperextension or Reverse Hyperextension (pages 85, 106–7)
- Dumbbell One-Arm Row (page 73)
- Cable Row (page 103)
- Dumbbell Hammer Curl (page 95)
- Shrug (page 81)

LAT PULLDOWN

- 1 set of 8 reps at medium weight
- 3 sets of 5 to 6 reps at heavy weight

T-BAR ROW

3 sets of 8 to 10 reps at heavy weight

DEADLIFT

- 1 set of 8 reps at light weight
- 1 set of 5 reps at medium to heavy weight
- 4 sets of 3 reps at heavy weight

BENT-OVER ROW

3 sets of 5 to 7 reps using heavy weight

CHIN-UP OR PULL-UP

3 sets of as many reps as possible

HYPEREXTENSION OR REVERSE HYPEREXTENSION

3 sets of 10 reps at body weight

DUMBBELL ONE-ARM ROW

3 sets of 6 to 10 reps using medium to heavy weight

CABLE ROW

3 sets of 8 to 10 reps with medium to heavy weight

DUMBBELL HAMMER CURL

3 sets of 8 to 10 reps using heavy dumbbells

SHRUG

Using a barbell or dumbbell, do 4 to 5 sets of 5 to 10 reps using heavy weight

DAY FOUR (legs, chest, triceps, and biceps)

WARM-UP: Stretch for 5 minutes. Do 2 sets of Hyperextensions, 10 reps each.

- Leg Press (page 109)
- Calf Raise Machine (pages 112–13)
- Bench Press (pages 56–57)
- Close-Grip Bench Press (page 68)
- Seated Press (page 69)
- Incline Bench Press (page 66)
- Lateral Raise (page 70)
- Triceps Lying Extension (page 90)
- Dip (page 77)
- Standing Barbell Curl (page 83)
- Dumbbell Hammer Curl (page 95)

LEG PRESS

- 1 set of 10 reps at 60 percent of body weight
- 4 sets of 5 to 6 reps at 80 percent of maximum leg-press weight

CALF RAISE MACHINE

3 sets of 8 to 10 reps at 85 percent of maximum leg-press weight

BENCH PRESS

- 1 set of 15 reps with just the bar
- 1 set of 10 reps at light weight
- 4 to 5 sets of 5 to 6 reps at 70 to 75 percent of maximum bench-press weight

CLOSE-GRIP BENCH PRESS

3 sets of 3 to 5 reps at 65 percent of maximum bench-press weight

SEATED PRESS

3 sets of 6 to 8 reps at medium to heavy dumbbell weight (bench should be at an eighty-degree angle)

DUMBBELL BENCH PRESS

2 to 3 sets of 8 to 10 reps at medium weight

INCLINE BENCH PRESS

2 to 3 sets of 6 to 8 reps using less weight than Dumbbell Bench Press

LATERAL RAISE

3 sets of 10 to 12 reps using light weight

TRICEPS LYING EXTENSION

1 set of 8 to 10 reps using light weight, then 3 sets of 6 reps at heavy weight

DIP

3 sets of 10 to 15 reps at body weight (when strength is built up, weight plates can be placed on legs for added resistance)

STANDING BARBELL CURL

3 sets of 8 to 10 reps at medium to heavy weight

DUMBBELL HAMMER CURL

3 sets of 5 to 6 reps using heavy dumbbells

CHAPTER 14
ADVANCED PROGRAM

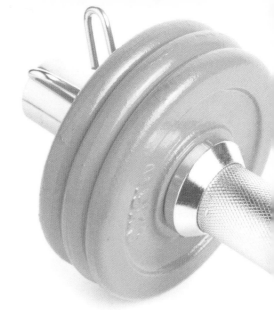

Continuing to improve and train at the advanced level requires incredible dedication. You won't meet your goals if you don't believe in yourself and your capabilities. You won't meet your goals if you miss workouts and get discouraged because the weights aren't increasing. At this stage of your strength and development, you'll have to begin experimenting with different techniques and methods for increasing your training proficiency.

This is a creative process we're outlining here that includes different levels to explore. The most intense workouts are the ones you want to focus all your energy on, and you'll have to perform with as much of a workload as you can tolerate, while still being able to recuperate after each session. This is where the "pure hard work" becomes purer and harder.

Stay motivated and determined. Above all, keep an open mind. By increasing your training volume and intensity, you'll be able to handle heavier weights for more sets and repetitions. The progression from beginner to intermediate to advanced involves months of work with medium to heavy resistance, and you'll be constantly pushing yourself to do more even as you think you've reached your limit. Slowly add a set here and a set there. In time you'll be able to perform and recuperate from immense workloads.

This could mean reaching your highest limits and goals with weights. Of course, this depends on how hard and long you want to stay strong and healthy. The more sophisticated your training becomes, the more it becomes a way of life. It's extremely difficult to reach your ultimate limit. Every year new training methods, lifting gear and equipment, and supplements can enhance an individual's ability to reach his ultimate limit. Barring injuries, men and women keep getting bigger, stronger, and more muscular. Usually when one hits a plateau one keeps training, but without the same intensity.

Your desire and motivation will make it impossible to even consider not going to the gym to train. The advanced athlete will believe that nothing on earth is as important to him as making that big lift. When you plan your workouts utilizing the Pure Hard Workout format, you'll feel a tremendous sense of accomplishment. You'll know that you've paid the price, and your effort and discipline have served you well. Nobody can train for you. Even when you're injured, beat up, or sore, you'll discover how your mind will motivate your body to overcome all obstacles. You must be determined to find a way to get to the top, like Tiki did.

The advanced athlete must have this mind-set. The way to develop perseverance is to learn to love your training. You won't develop any real size or strength without learning to love the hard work, making the effort, and feeling the pain, muscle aches, and pounding in your head. You must learn to love the workout no matter how demanding it becomes. But if you're determined to build yourself up and overcome poor genetics or poor health, then nothing will interfere with you reaching your goals.

DAY ONE (legs and abdominals)

WARM-UP: Stretch for 10 minutes, then 2 sets of Hyperextensions of 15 reps each

- Leg Press (page 109)
- Calf Raise Machine (pages 112–13)
- Front Squat (page 70)
- Squat (pages 54–55)
- Hack Squat or Leg Extension (pages 108, 110)
- Stiff-Legged Deadlift or Leg Curl (pages 63, 111)
- Good Morning (page 84)
- Reverse Hyperextension (pages 106–7)
- Plank Hold (page 129)
- Hanging Leg Raise (page 120)
- Dumbbell Side Bend (page 125)

LEG PRESS

- 1 set of 10 reps at 55 percent of maximum leg-press weight
- 1 set of 5 reps at 75 percent of maximum leg-press weight
- 4 sets of 2 to 3 reps at 87 percent of maximum leg-press weight

CALF RAISE MACHINE

4 sets of 5 to 6 reps using heavy weight

FRONT SQUAT

- 4 sets of 3 to 5 reps at 50 percent of maximum weight
- 1 set of 5 reps at 70 percent of maximum weight
- 4 sets of 2 to 3 reps at 86 percent of maximum weight

SQUAT

- 2 sets of 10 reps at 50 percent of maximum weight
- 1 set of 5 reps at 70 percent of maximum weight
- 4 sets of 2 to 3 reps at 86 percent of maximum weight

HACK SQUAT OR LEG EXTENSION

2 sets of 10 reps using medium to heavy weight

STIFF-LEGGED DEADLIFT OR LEG CURL

3 sets of 8 to 10 reps

GOOD MORNING

3 sets of 3 to 5 reps: 1 light set and 2 heavier sets

REVERSE HYPEREXTENSION

3 sets of 8 to 10 reps at medium to heavy weight

PLANK HOLD

3 sets of 10 to 15 reps

HANGING LEG RAISE

3 sets of 10 to 20 reps at body weight

DUMBBELL SIDE BEND

3 sets of 10 to 12 reps

Note: This is also a good day to pull or drag a weighted sled for cardio and recuperation.

DAY TWO (chest, triceps, waist, and forearms)

WARM-UP: Stretch for 10 minutes. Do 2 sets of Hyperextensions of 15 reps each.

- Bench Press (page 56-57)
- Incline Bench Press (page 66)
- Close-Grip Bench Press (page 68)
- Dip (page 77)
- Dumbbell Fly (page 71)
- Dumbbell Pullover (page 72)
- Triceps Pushdown (page 105)
- Triceps Lying Extension (page 90)
- Triceps Dumbbell Kickback (page 91)
- Side Sit-up
- Arms Overhead Sit-up
- Leg Raise (Lying: page 119; Hanging: page 120)
- Wrist Roller (page 114)
- Standing Wrist Curl (page 98)
- Plate-Loaded Grip (page 115)

BENCH PRESS

- 1 set of 20 reps with just the bar
- 1 set of 10 reps at light weight
- 1 set of 6 reps at 65 percent of maximum bench-press weight
- 4 to 5 sets of 1 to 2 reps at 88 to 90 percent of maximum bench-press weight

INCLINE BENCH PRESS

3 sets of 5 to 6 reps at heavy weight

CLOSE-GRIP BENCH PRESS

3 sets of 6 reps at 65 percent maximum bench-press weight

DIP

Using a Dip belt, do 3 sets of 3 to 5 reps, adding weight to the belt for increased resistance

DUMBBELL FLY

3 sets of 8 to 10 reps at medium weight (you may also occasionally do Dumbbell Flys on an incline or decline bench)

DUMBBELL PULLOVER

3 to 4 sets of 8 to 10 reps (build slowly to heavy weights)

TRICEPS PUSHDOWN

3 to 4 sets of 6 to 8 reps at heavy weight

TRICEPS LYING EXTENSION

4 sets of 8 to 10 reps using heavy weight

TRICEPS DUMBBELL KICKBACK

3 sets of 8 to 10 reps using medium to heavy weight

SIDE SIT-UP

3 sets of 10 to 15 reps at body weight

ARMS OVERHEAD SIT-UP

3 sets of 10 to 15 reps using light resistance

LEG RAISE

3 sets of 8 to 10 reps using medium to heavy resistance

WRIST ROLLER

Roll the rope up and down 3 times using good resistance

STANDING WRIST CURL

3 sets of 5 to 7 reps using heavy weight

PLATE-LOADED GRIP

3 times medium-heavy weight, max reps

DAY THREE (shoulders and abs)

WARM-UP: Stretch for 10 minutes. Do 2 sets of Hyperextensions of 15 reps each.

- Shoulder Press Machine (page 101)
- Military Press
- Upright Row (page 80)
- Bent-Over Lateral (page 78)
- Front Dumbbell Raise (page 88)
- Shrug (page 81)
- Standing Barbell Curl (page 83)
- Dumbbell Hammer Curl (page 95)
- Power Hold (page 96)
- Russian Twist (page 123)
- Windmill (page 126)
- Medicine Ball Work (page 122)

SHOULDER PRESS MACHINE

- 2 sets with light weight
- 1 set of 5 reps using medium to heavy weight
- 3 to 4 sets of 4 to 5 reps each, using heavy weight

MILITARY PRESS

3 sets of 6 reps using medium to heavy weight

UPRIGHT ROW

3 sets of 8 reps using medium to heavy weight

BENT-OVER LATERAL

3 sets of 8 to 10 reps using medium to heavy weight

FRONT DUMBBELL RAISE

2 sets of 8 to 10 reps using heavy weight

SHRUG

Using a barbell or dumbbells, do 4 sets of 5 to 7 reps using medium to heavy weight

STANDING BARBELL CURL

4 sets of 3 to 5 reps using heavy weight

DUMBBELL HAMMER CURL

3 sets of 5 to 7 reps using heavy weight

POWER HOLD

3 times using heavy weight

RUSSIAN TWIST

3 sets of 10 to 15 reps at medium weight

WINDMILL

3 sets of 15 to 20 reps

MEDICINE BALL WORK

3 sets of 10 to 12 reps

DAY FOUR (back and biceps)

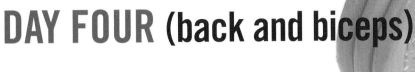

WARM-UP: Stretch for 10 minutes. Do 2 sets of Hyperextensions of 15 reps each.

- Lat Pulldown (page 100)
- T-Bar Row (page 104)
- Deadlift (pages 59–61)
- Deadlift Off Box (page 62)
- Power Clean (pages 86–87)
- Bent-Over Row (page 74)
- Dumbbell One-Arm Row (page 73)
- Chin-up or Pull-up (pages 75–76)
- Shrug (page 81)
- Hyperextension (page 85)
- Standing Barbell Curl (page 83)
- Preacher Curl (page 94)
- Dumbbell Hammer Curl (page 95)
- Sled Work (or Sandbag Work)

LAT PULLDOWN

3 sets of 8 reps using medium to heavy weight (pull to front)

T-BAR ROW

3 sets of 8 reps, using medium to heavy weight

DEADLIFT

2 light warm-ups, followed by 4 sets of 3 reps each at 85 percent of maximum Deadlift weight

DEADLIFT OFF BOX

2 to 3 sets of 3 reps using less weight than a regular Deadlift

POWER CLEAN

4 sets of 2 to 3 reps at medium to heavy weight

BENT-OVER ROW

3 sets of 5 to 7 reps at medium to heavy weight

DUMBBELL ONE-ARM ROW

3 sets of 6 reps using heavy weight

CHIN-UP OR PULL-UP

3 reps, though number will vary with each individual (you can also use a lat machine with an underhand grip, similar to a regular Chin-up)

SHRUG

4 to 5 sets of 6 to 8 reps using heavy weights

HYPEREXTENSION

3 sets of 10 reps, using body weight for added resistance

STANDING BARBELL CURL

3 sets of 6 to 8 reps using heavy weight

PREACHER CURL

3 sets of 8 to 10 reps using medium to heavy weight

DUMBBELL HAMMER CURL

Using heavy dumbbells, do 3 sets of 5 to 7 reps

SLED WORK (OR SANDBAG WORK)

Pulling and dragging

DAY FIVE (legs and chest)

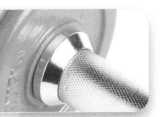

WARM-UP: Stretch for 10 minutes. Do 2 sets of Hyperextensions of 15 reps each.

- Leg Press (page 109)
- Front Squat (page 70)
- Bench Press (pages 56–57)
- Incline Bench Press (page 66)
- Close-Grip Bench Press (page 68)
- Dumbbell Fly (page 71)
- Dumbbell Pullover (page 72)

LEG PRESS

1 set of 10 reps using 55 percent of maximum leg-press weight

FRONT SQUAT

1 set of 10 reps at light weight, followed by 3 sets of 5 to 8 reps at 70 percent intensity

BENCH PRESS

- 1 set of 10 to 15 reps at light weight
- 4 sets of 3 to 5 reps at 80 to 85 percent of maximum bench-press weight

INCLINE BENCH PRESS

3 sets of 6 to 7 reps at medium to heavy weight

CLOSE-GRIP BENCH PRESS

3 sets of 4 to 5 reps at 75 percent of maximum bench-press weight

DUMBBELL FLY

3 sets of 6 to 8 reps at medium to heavy weight

DUMBBELL PULLOVER

2 sets of 10 reps at medium to heavy weight

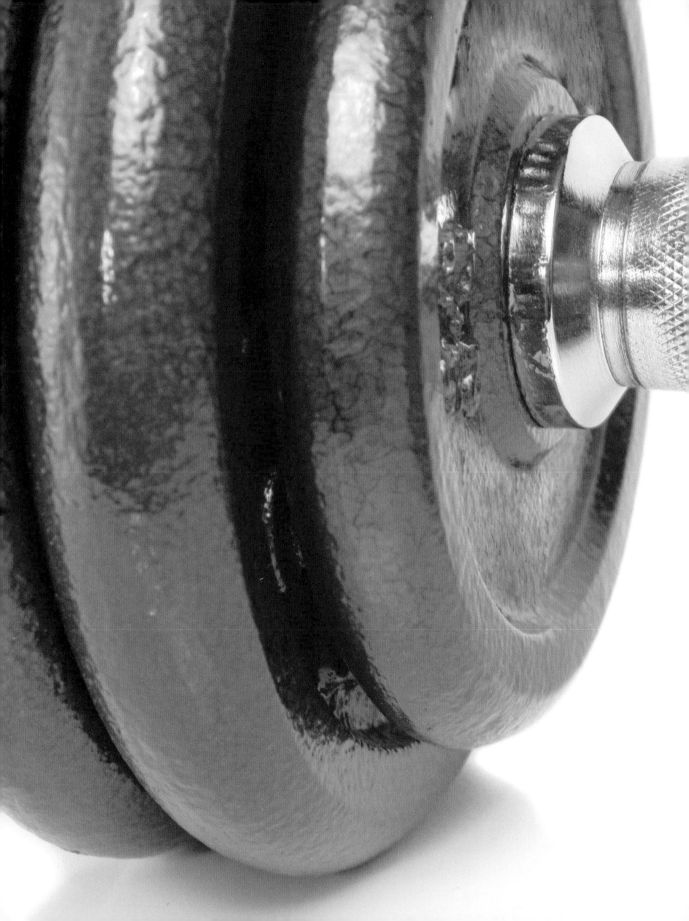

THE THREE-DAYS-PER-WEEK WORKOUT

You have to train smart if your time is limited. The smartest move is to *always do the big lifts first*. For instance, don't do sets of dumbbell lateral raises for your shoulders before military presses. Kill yourself first with heavy military presses, then do a few lighter sets of lateral raises. These won't build your shoulders up like military presses will.

Whether you're starting a beginner, intermediate, or advanced program, you'll get maximum results by following it to the letter. However, if you're struggling with time constraints, then on day one just do Squats and Bench Presses. On day two, do a shoulder workout, if that's all you have time for. On day three concentrate on Deadlifts and maybe Bent-Over Rows. You'll still get big and strong doing just these three power lifts. You can do your main lift for a particular workout and your assistance work the following day. You'll also gain body weight because you'll be building in time to recuperate.

If you're focusing on size and strength and you have only about three hours per week to work out, you should carve out time for three 1-hour sessions every other day, as follows:

DAY ONE: Monday

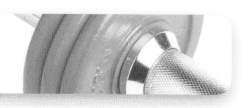

WARM-UP: Stretch for 5 minutes.

CORE LIFTS

Squat (pages 54–55): 5 sets, 3–5 reps, using 70–85 percent of your maximum load

Leg Press (page 109): 3 sets, 6 reps, using heavy weight

Bench Press (page 56–57): 5 sets, 3–5 reps, using 70–85 percent of your maximum load

Sit-up (page 118): 2–3 sets, 15–25 reps with resistance

VARIATIONS

Dip (page 77): 3 sets, 5–7 reps, with additional weight

Close-Grip Bench Press (page 68): 3–4 sets, 5–7 reps, using medium weight

Barbell Curl (page 83): 3 sets, 8–10 reps

DAY TWO: Wednesday

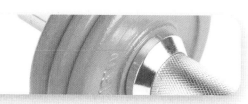

WARM-UP: 5-minute stretch

CORE LIFTS

Military Press (page 58): 5 sets, 3–5 reps, with heavy weight

Seated Dumbbell Press (page 69): 3 sets, 5–7 reps, with heavy weight

Upright Row (page 80): 3 sets, 6–8 reps, with just enough weight to still maintain good form

Leg Raise (Lying: page 119; Hanging: page 120): 2–3 sets, 15–25 reps

VARIATIONS

Bent-Over Lateral (page 78): 3 sets, 8–10 reps, with just enough weight to still maintain good form

Shrug (page 81): 5 sets, 5–7 reps, with heavy weight

Triceps Lying Extension (page 90): 4 sets, 8–10 reps

Dumbbell Hammer Curl (page 95): 3 sets, 5–8 reps, with heavy weight

ASSISTED MOVEMENTS

Triceps Pushdown (page 105): 4 sets, 6–8 reps, with heavy weight

DAY THREE: Friday

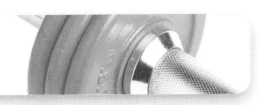

WARM-UP: Stretch for 5 minutes.

CORE LIFTS

Deadlift (pages 59–61): 5 sets, 3–5 reps, building up to heavy weight

Bent-Over Row (page 74): 3 sets, 5–8 reps, with heavy weight

VARIATIONS

Shrug (page 81): 3 sets, 10 reps, with heavy weight

Standing Barbell Curl (page 83): 3 sets, 8–10 reps

Standing Wrist Curl (page 98): 3 sets, 10 reps, with medium weight

ASSISTED MOVEMENTS

Lat Pulldown (page 100): 3 sets, 8–10 reps, with medium weight

Knee Lift on a Dip Stand (page 121): 3 sets, 15–20 reps

This schedule will give you a great 3-hour-per-week workout. It works every body part hard and, in some cases, more than once. If you're short on time, concentrate on the core lifts and one or two variations, and you'll finish in one hour. If time permits, you can always throw in an extra exercise of your choice. Consider Calf Raises or an extra set or two to work your weak areas—e.g., Dumbbell Pullovers for your chest. And remember: No talking during the workout, just pure hard work.

CHAPTER 15
WILLPOWER MEETS HEAVY LIFTING

T oo many athletes and coaches ignore such tools as sandbags, logs, anvils, and sled dragging during their workouts. These can dramatically help develop a person's strength and power just as much, if not more, than your standard free weights. Strongman workouts are an ideal way to improve your overall muscular development as well as build up your athletic skills, range of motion, flexibility, strength, and endurance. In short, they'll turn you into a beast.

There are no set rules for deciding when you're physically ready for this type of training. Before moving to Strongman training, try cutting down your rest time between free weight sets. Many athletes think they need all day to rest between heavy sets. This isn't the case. Or they believe that extra conditioning will mess up their heavy workouts. Wrong. They're just not in good enough shape to go from one heavy set to the next.

The better conditioned you are, the faster your recovery will be. Poor conditioning, on

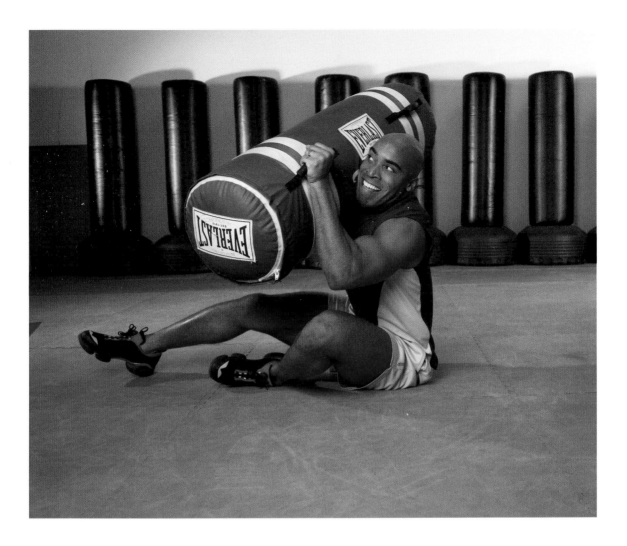

the other hand, will leave you unable to hit the weights hard, and this will only encourage failure and disappointment.

Strongman cardio exercises can be employed at the end of your regular workout. Because these are excellent for overall strength and conditioning, they could replace some of your regular cardio work if you do them, say, three to five times per week. They will definitely complement both your cardio routines and your strength training.

Say you live in an area whose climate forces you to do your cardio work indoors during some seasons. Grab a pair of dumbbells and do the Farmer's Walk, or improvise weight-carrying exercises that work on your cardio conditioning. You can change your routines every two to three weeks so you won't get bored. You'll really be able to push yourself this way.

It's very important to gradually build these exercises into your regular workouts. Pushing yourself beyond your limits will only slow you down, so make sure you set a deliberate pace and stick to it. Your goal should be one strongman cardio exercise per workout, but start off by doing one per week. Use light weights of 10 to 20 pounds, and go a short distance. Slowly work your way up until you're walking or running for longer distances. When the fixed weight becomes too easy, add more.

You should always strive for new heights, but ultimately only you can judge that threshold; whether it's two weeks, a month, or even a few months. It can be a humbling experience to try to push yourself to the maximum of your abilities. You'll feel a burn in your chest and muscles that you've never felt before, and eventually you'll come to enjoy this burn. When you can handle three or four days per week of strongman cardio, you'll really start reaping the benefits. As your cardiovascular system becomes more conditioned and your entire body strengthens, your weight workouts will be much more efficient. You'll start seeing the snowball effect, when each workout strengthens you and allows you to lift more and push more.

Of course, strongman cardio does put extra stress on knee and ankle joints. If you have previous injuries, you must pay close attention to them and build up very slowly. Make sure you alleviate the stress on injured areas with stretching and cold packs after your workout. Walking or running with weights can be very therapeutic for injuries if you take your time and build up gradually.

And obviously, we don't recommend this for people who are so out of shape that they can't walk up stairs without huffing and puffing. These exercisers will want to start with simple walking, gradually adding an incline, and even more gradually, light weights. Beginners should be able to carry on a conversation while performing cardio work.

If you're healthy and have no prior injuries to your knees or ankles, running or walking with weights will not only build up tremendous tendon, cartilage, and ligament strength, but also whole-body strength. Lifters of all different body weights, who are in fairly good condition, will enjoy strongman cardio because it's a great break from heavy weight training. After a backbreaking workout, these exercises will help with recovery.

SANDBAGS AND HEAVY, AWKWARD OBJECTS

Lifting sandbags and heavy, awkward objects such as logs, anvils, and barrels is not for the fainthearted. This is a whole different animal from lifting barbells and dumbbells. Sandbags and anvils are *a lot* harder to control.

Consider a straight clean-and-press with a barbell. No problem, right? Try this with a hundred-plus-pound bag filled with shifting sand, forcing you to fight for control. This becomes a total-body exercise. The same is true for kegs, barrels, and steel beams.

The hardest weight to lift is awkward weight because it puts stress on all the big, powerful muscles, from all angles, and also brings into play all the stabilizer muscles or smaller muscle groups, for example, the lower back, ankles, knees, wrists, and elbows.

SANDBAG TRAINING

The sandbag works the body in ways barbells, dumbbells, or weight machines can't. It reaches muscle areas that can't be reached with conventional equipment. Tiki had to manhandle a bag weighing more than 130 pounds using sheer power. He developed great overall body strength and a good grip for holding on to the football. He also built up in three other key areas: the stabilizers in his upper back, which help support his arms while lifting heavy weights overhead; the obliques, which help support his abdomen and back muscles during Squats and Deadlifts; and the ankles and calf muscles, which help support his legs during Squats. In addition to the bag, he used steel logs to develop the rugged power required in football and other physical contact sports.

Ideally, you should construct a couple of sandbags of different sizes and weights. This will allow you to use the one that's best suited for a particular exercise, number of repetitions, or workout. If you're strong and in really good condition, use heavier sandbags ranging from 70 to 125 pounds. If you're just beginning your training, start with sandbags ranging from 25 to 50 pounds. Some exercises are more difficult than others and require less weight for more effective sandbag training.

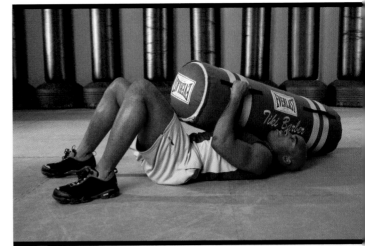

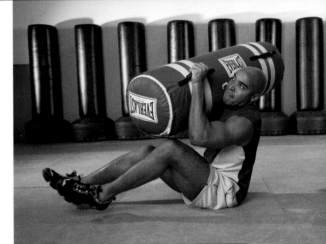

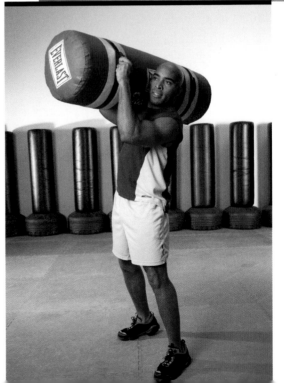

For example, Sandbag Curls, Sandbag Presses, and Overhead Sandbag Front Raises, all require less weight than Sandbag Squats, Sandbag Deadlifts, Sandbag Bear Hugs, or just shouldering the sandbag and walking with it. For endurance training, consider 8 to 10 repetitions of the exercise using lighter bags. For building muscle strength, do 6 repetitions with the heavy bags. Be sure, though, to train at your own pace because these exercises will work you, and work you hard.

One of the best things to do with a sandbag is to start lying on the ground with the bag on your chest. Simply try to get up and get the bag on your shoulder, any way you can.

The strongman exercises are particularly useful for wrestlers, football players, and other athletes who use their hands and fingers when battling in their respective sports. Hand and finger strength is a great asset and can give you a tremendous advantage over your opponents.

It's important to keep your back straight when you're squatting, deadlifting, or doing barbell rows to prevent injury and build back strength. However, when you pick up a heavy sandbag, anvil, or keg filled with sand or water, you really have to do it with a rounded back. This helps build your lower back and side muscles, as well as improve your grip and forearm strength.

Hefting these objects builds tremendous body power and endurance. It also toughens your mind and tests your willpower. It takes years of hard, progressive exercise to build up

your physical endurance. Regardless of if you use sandbags or heavy stones, it's still pure hard work.

SLEDGEHAMMER WORK

As previously mentioned, the most difficult type of weight to lift is an awkward one or any weight that's held away from the body, mostly because it puts maximum stress on the

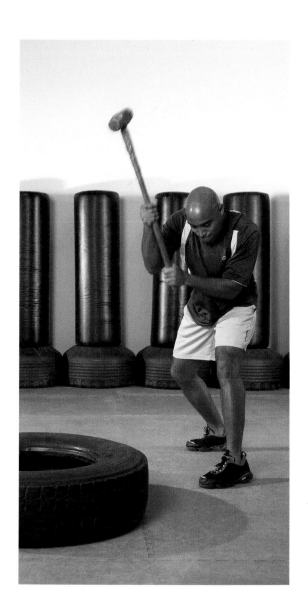

muscles from severe angles. A sledgehammer fits right into this category.

When the weight is in front of your body, it stresses all the muscles in your backside, feet, and calves. When the weight is to the side, it stresses the waist, thighs, and hips. When the weight is behind you, it works your stomach, front thighs, and chest. When you raise the weight overhead, it taxes all your upper-body muscles. When you swing the weight from front to back, you're working all your twisting muscles. The sledgehammer is great for an athlete in any sport or for any person interested in developing strength, coordination, and stamina. Of course, you'll need to find a sturdy sledgehammer of 9 to 10 pounds. Tiki would beat on an old truck tire, but you can swing against any surface that will soften the blow.

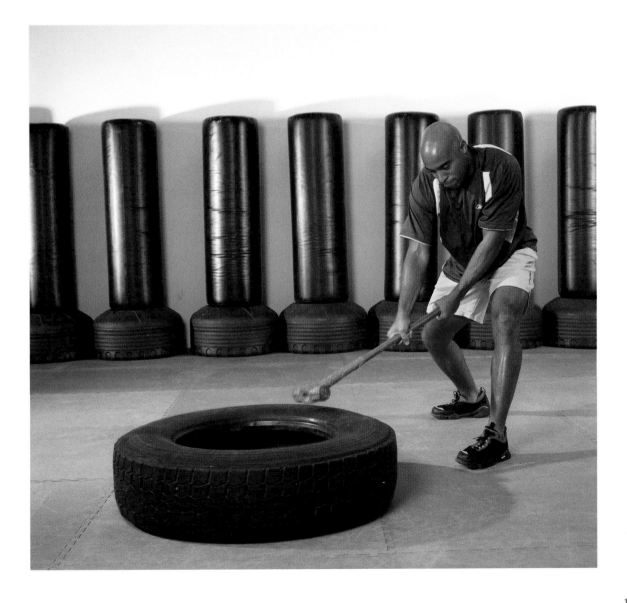

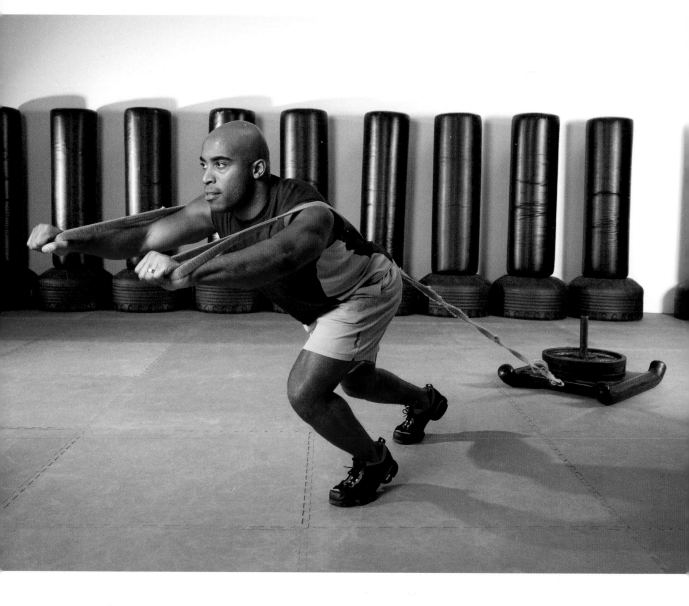

SLED TRAINING

Sled dragging has become popular, particularly with powerlifters, football players, and professional fighters. It offers versatility and low impact. Dragging provides an easy way to load almost any muscle group while virtually eliminating the stressful, eccentric component responsible for delayed-onset muscle soreness. Sled dragging is ideal for condition-ing workouts during periods of heavy lifting or sports training. It can also be used effectively as a recovery workout to flush out sore muscles.

This exercise involves a piece of exercise equipment with a welded-steel sled equipped with a harness and/or handles that provide endless pushing or dragging variations. Using a sled is a great way to enhance speed strength and strength speed. You can load up the sled with light weights or heavy weights. To use any significant weight, you have to lean forward at the waist until your shoulders are at about the same level as your hips, and you're driving the effort through your feet.

The first couple of steps are the hardest. As you build momentum, you'll notice a tendency to let your upper body rise. This will make the work more difficult and transfer the workload from the quadriceps to the hamstrings. Each step should be quick and short. Concentrate on keeping your shoulders low, and continue pushing on your toes.

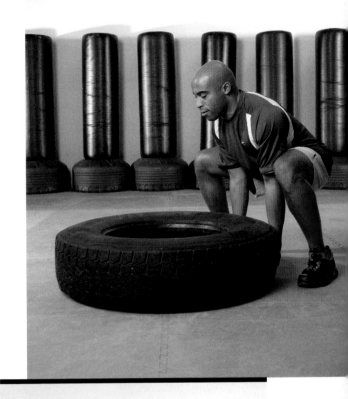

TIRE FLIPPING

Tire flipping is similar to deadlifting in that it places demand on your legs and lower-back muscles. You start by wedging your hands under a tire, and driving up with your legs and back until the tire is at about shoulder height. From this position, you push forward explosively with your entire body to tip it over. Tire flips can be done for distance, reps, or time intervals.

TRUCK PUSHING

All you need is a truck (the bigger the better), and some willpower for this one—Shaun O'Hara of the Giants was kind enough to lend us his Hummer. Find an empty paved surface, throw the truck into neutral, and start pushing. To make it harder, you can push it up a slight incline. Just make sure you have someone in the driver's seat to hit the brake if necessary!

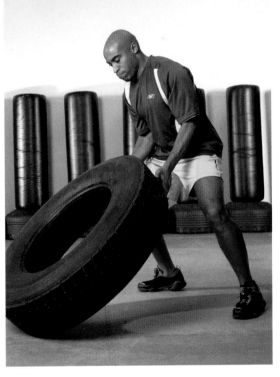

TRUCK PUSHING

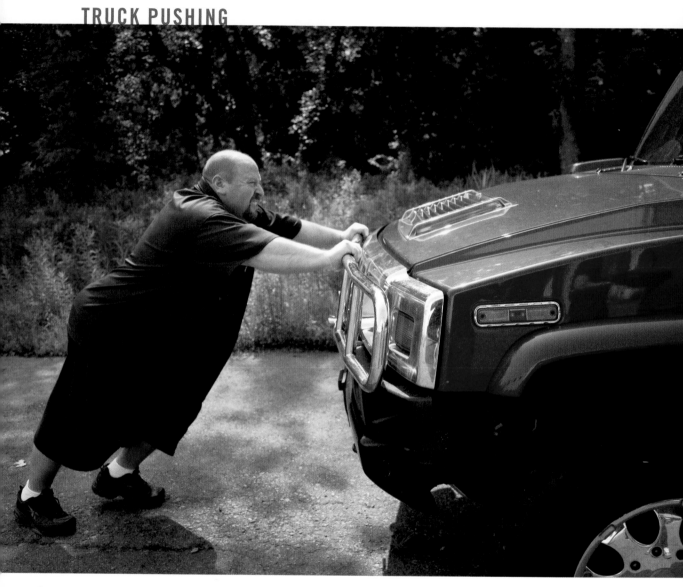

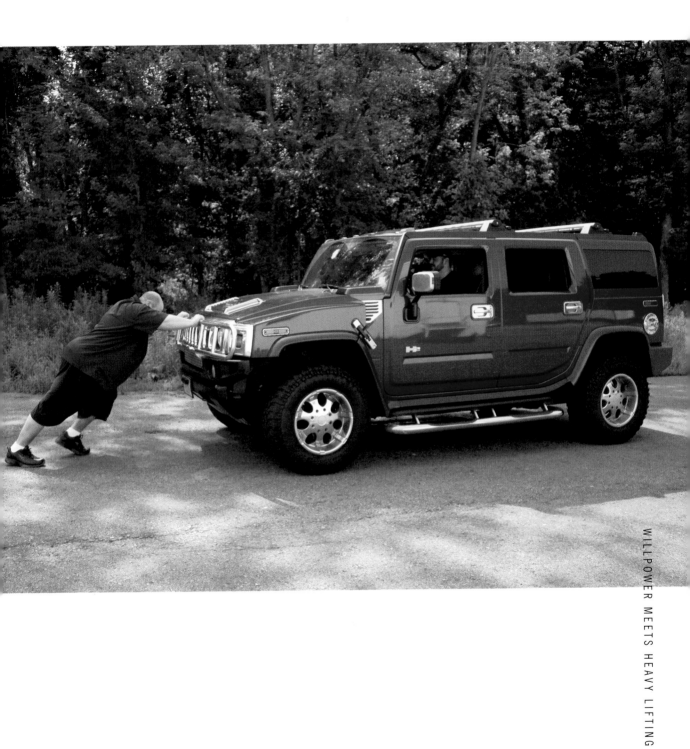

One of the things that Tiki enjoyed from these exercises was breaking away from our traditional regimen of working predominantly with a barbell or dumbbells. The routines made Tiki strong all over. In his final regular-season game, a defender attempted to "horse-collar" tackle Tiki. Because Tiki was stronger, he broke through the tackle, but the defender fell with all of his weight on Tiki's ankle. For a sickening second, Tiki feared it was broken. However, he flexed it and discovered it was fine. When Tiki told me this, I could only respond, "Good thing you've been Canini-ized!"

WALKING WITH WEIGHTS

Carrying weight is the true measure of strength. Whether it's a rock carried at waist or chest level, or a barbell across the shoulders, walking with heavy weight builds tremendous endurance, strength, and coordination. It also develops your ankles, shins, calves, and thighs; the front and sides of your stomach, and lower and upper back; and your shoulders, chest, hands, wrists, arms, and neck. Use weight that's just heavy enough to make you slightly winded at the end of each set. A set should be 25 steps.

These are all great conditioners and strength builders. There are numerous ways to use common gym equipment to accomplish similar goals. The ones mentioned below should stimulate some creative ideas of your own.

FARMER'S WALK

This is a terrific overall body movement, provided that your grip is strong enough to handle heavy poundage. Find two weights of equal size (two dumbbells or two steel pipes with handles), get a good grip, and take a walk while holding your chest high and the weights down by your sides. You can walk for distance or for time. If you go for distance, try to walk between 50 and 100 yards. For time, try to go a few minutes at a time.

OVERHEAD WALK

This is a technique that Joe learned from trainer John Davies. Simply take a weight and carry it overhead for a certain time or distance. Mix it up to stay motivated. Use a barbell for one routine, and a dumbbell for the next.

BAR CARRY

Load up a barbell with approximately 30 to 45 percent of your squatting weight. Place the bar on your back and begin walking. The more turns you can make, the more challenging the drill will be on the core muscles. If you're using dumbbells, you can carry one in front of your body, cradling it near your chest, or carry two in a Hammer Curl grip. You'll

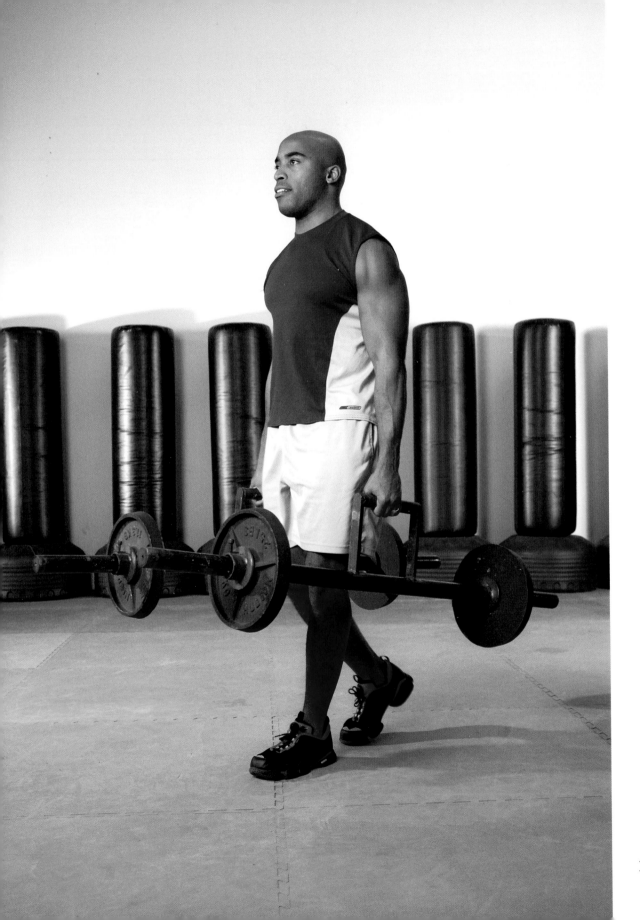

THE TIKI BAG
AND YOKE

The bag I designed for Tiki enabled me to develop a unique way of strengthening his body from head to toe. Our friend Adam Gesler, from the Everlast sporting goods company, had it specially made for us.

The bag looks like the everyday heavy bag used by boxers, only I had special handles placed in different locations. This enabled Tiki to grab it from any angle. I invented this bag for Tiki initially because he wanted to improve his pass-blocking skills. Every year we'd evaluate his previous season. Tiki got the ball in nearly half of the plays, but on those that he didn't, he had to block. The 130-pound Tiki bag worked just the way I thought it would: It built tremendous toughness and fierce determination in Tiki. I'd have him lie on his back, and then direct him to stand up with the bag on his shoulders without using his hands.

Using the bag, we did Power Cleans, Squats, and agility drills. These exercises worked all of the pulling muscles, including the trunk and hips. Walking with the bag strengthened his lower back, hips, and knees, which enabled him to break tackles. Tiki also did these exercises using the yoke—a heavy frame that fits over the shoulders and on which additional weights can be hung at either end. The yoke helped with Tiki's balance. Alone it weighed 230 pounds, and we often added up to 420 pounds. Tiki carried it a distance of 20 to 30 yards and then turned around and walked back. Sometimes I'd have him walk sideways like a carioca dancer. He'd move like this for 10 to 20 yards.

When we completed the yoke carries, I would have Tiki get under the yoke and do quarter squats. The great thing about these movements is they build great tendon strength and toughen the body for full-range movements. In partial movements you can use a lot more weight than you can in full-range movements because you're not moving the weight as far.

Still other items Tiki and I used to build his overall strength and body power were logs weighing 135 pounds and 170 pounds. The handles were parallel to the body instead of perpendicular, which made picking them up and power cleaning them much more difficult than using a 45-pound Olympic bar.

This type of training builds great shoulder and triceps strength. In addition, it builds trapezius strength when you're pressing the log overhead. The steel logs are more than 8 feet in length, and they're difficult to clean and press overhead. They're great, though, for strengthening the stabilizers of the back and shoulders. Tiki attacked the steel logs aggressively, and I was pleased with his commitment to conquer all different forms of training techniques.

—JOE

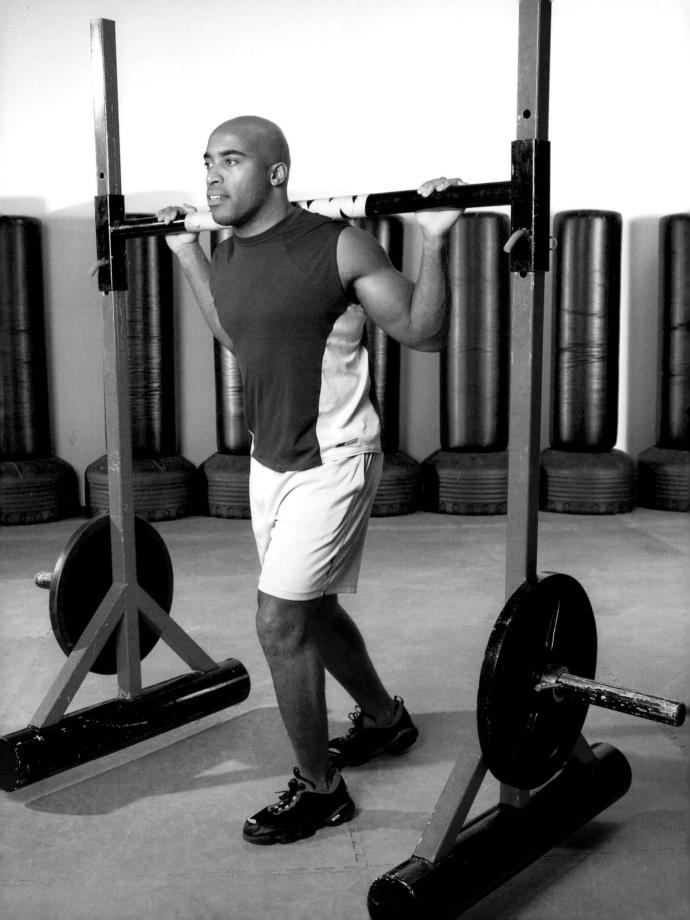

discover whole new muscle groups in your back and upper body. Plate carries can be performed in the same manner.

DEADLIFT CARRY

Choose a load that you can hold for 30 seconds. Deadlift the weight to a standing position and begin to walk in various directions. You can choose distance, time, or a certain number of repetitions per exercise, or simply continue until you're completely fatigued.

Whether you're lifting and working out with heavy sandbags, carrying heavy stones, pushing a four-ton truck, or pushing cars, you must have good wind and endurance. Nothing works better at building endurance than these demanding tests of strength. As you advance in your training, it's a good idea to do some unusual exercises to develop all-around strength. This kind of training strengthens the body and toughens the mind.

The harder you push yourself during these workouts, the easier the more typical workouts will become. Remember that consistency—one good workout after the other—is key to success in the world of strength. You can build muscle strength by itself, but you won't get the most out of it if you don't build up your endurance and health, too.

CHAPTER 16
WOMEN AND WEIGHTLIFTING

T hrough the sensible use of weight training, thousands of women who've never considered themselves athletic are turning shapeless bodies into firm, toned, and healthy ones. The past thirty years have shown an increase in women's awareness of the value of working out with weights. More women are using weights and finding that the benefits of regular weight training aren't simply cosmetic as previously believed.

In some cases women will benefit from *adding* body weight rather than losing it. This isn't weight in the form of useless fat, but rather healthy, solid, contoured muscle. Keep in mind that women who train with weights won't develop rippling muscles or the clear-cut defini-tion of male bodybuilders because women don't have the genetic makeup or hormones that pro-duce or allow muscular bulk like men. The ad-ditional layer of body fat on most women hides the muscular separation, but allows female muscle to show off as graceful curves.

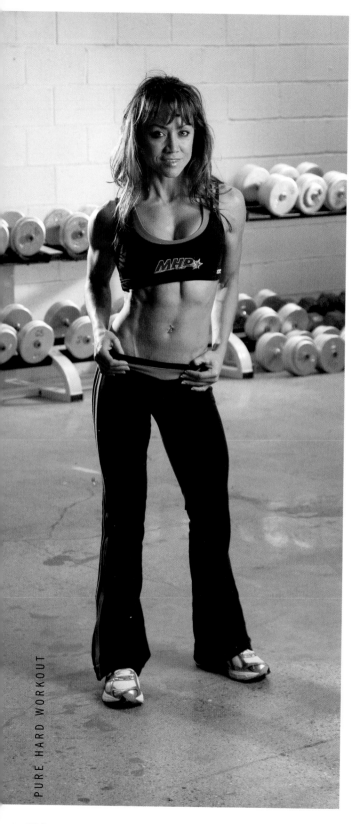

Although going to the gym can provide a pleasant atmosphere, it doesn't help to alter the shape of your body if you're sticking to the elliptical machine and yoga classes. As with men, the key is dumbbells, barbells, and weight machines. Before signing up with one of those glamorous gyms, be sure it has the essential equipment required to get a full-body workout.

TRAINING AT HOME

Home training can be especially suitable for women because their training doesn't require the same heavy equipment as that of men. If you have only the odd half hour or hour to spare, then home training is ideal. Health-conscious couples will often exercise together. Here again, the home gym or home training is ideal and can be more effective than a professional gym.

The first requirement for home training is a set of weights. The set doesn't have to be as heavy as the ones designed for men. Start off with dumbbells of equal weight. You can begin with 2 to 3 pounds and 5 to 10 pounds. Another suggestion would be to consider purchasing an exercise bench and an abdominals board. Remember that these can be improvised; it's not necessary to buy anything too costly or fancy. Women can use less expensive versions of the same basic type of weights and benches that men use.

EXERCISES FOR A FULL-BODY WORKOUT

When planning your schedule, consider these exercises. They're the same ones that men use to increase muscle strength, but you won't have to do as many reps of each exercise, or use weights as heavy, to achieve the effect you want. You'll want to work the entire body, so execute exercises for each body part. As with any new program, pay attention to how your body "talks back" after a workout, and adjust the intensity accordingly. You don't ever want to be so stiff that you can't work out the next day.

- Bench Press
- Dumbbell Bench Press
- Bent-Arm Pullover
- Chair Dip
- Dumbbell Fly
- Incline Bench Press
- Squat
- Lunge
- Leg Extension
- Leg Curl
- Calf Raise
- Leg Split

In general, you'll do the same exercises as the men. Below are some exercises that women may particularly benefit from, however.

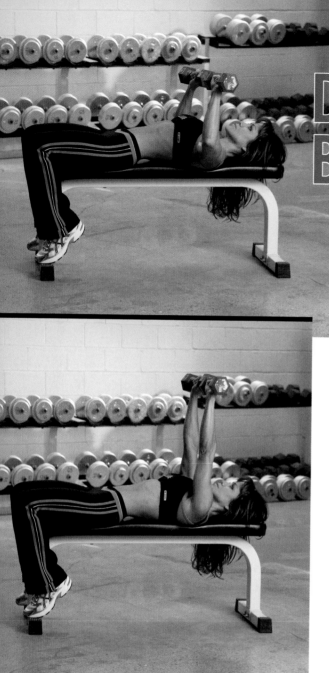

DUMBBELL BENCH PRESS

MUSCLE GROUP: pectorals

SETUP:

Lie on the bench.

Take a comfortable grip on a pair of dumbbells and hold them above your chest at arm's length.

STEP ONE: Lower the weights until your elbows are at a ninety-degree angle or until they touch the center of your chest.

STEP TWO: Forcefully extend the dumbbells over your chest.

Tiki Tip: Vary your grip on the dumbbells. Try hands in a vertical position every few workouts for variety.

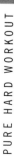

DUMBBELL FLY

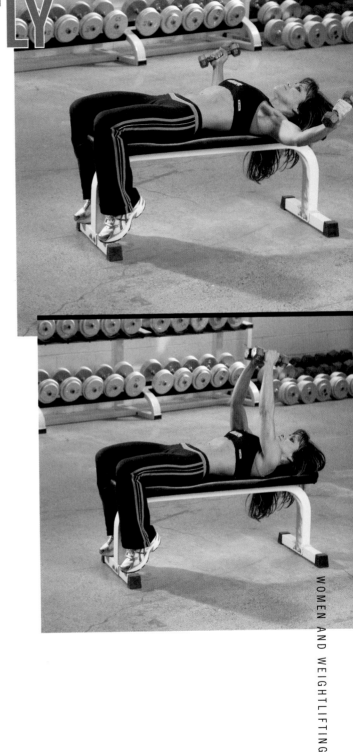

MUSCLE GROUP: pectorals

SETUP:

Lie on a bench on your back with two dumbbells held at arm's length above the shoulders.

STEP ONE: Breathe in deeply as you slowly swing your arms in a downward arc so that they end up extended away from your body. Unlock the arms slightly as you lower them.

STEP TWO: Return to the starting point, exhaling as you do so and keeping the arms just off lock until the last few inches, when they may be straightened.

Tiki Tip: Again, like the Dumbbell Bench Press, this one is particularly suited to ladies.

BENCH DIP

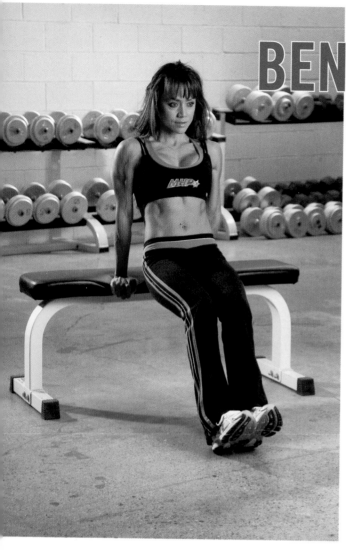

MUSCLE GROUP: deltoids, triceps, and pectorals

SETUP:

Place your hands on the seat of a bench behind you.

Bend your legs at the knees, forming a right angle, and balance. Find a stable point that's comfortable.

Push yourself up until your arms are locked straight and you're supporting your weight with your arm and shoulder muscles. Remain in this position, holding your body weight.

STEP ONE: Bend your arms, allowing your body to lower toward the floor.

STEP TWO: Push yourself back to the starting position, exhaling as you do so.

Tiki Tip: In its ordinary form as Push-ups, most women find that they're unable to do sufficient, if any, repetitions in decent style. The Chair Dip is different. Anybody can manage this and get great results if they keep at it.

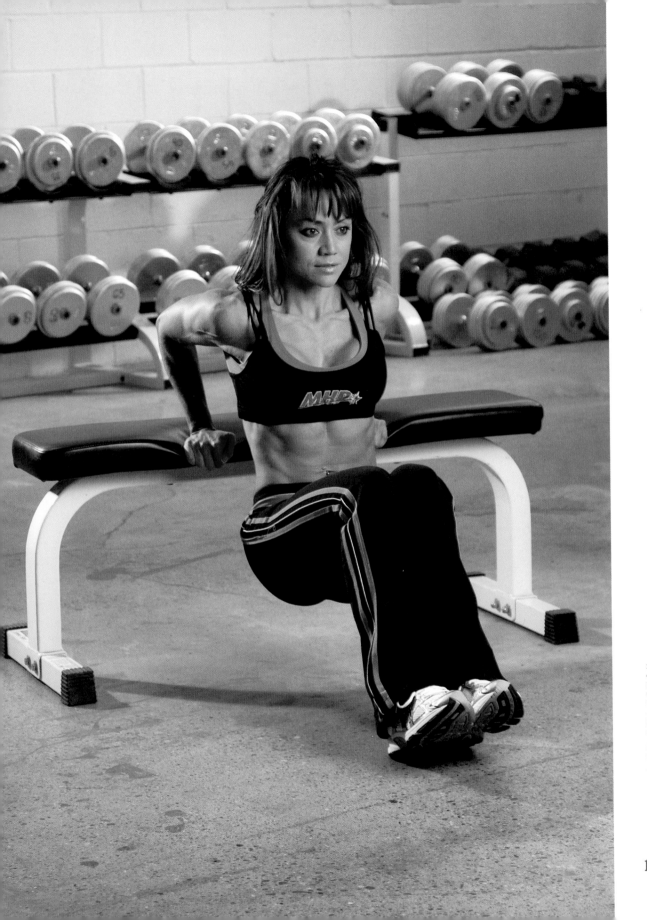

WOMEN AND WEIGHTLIFTING

189

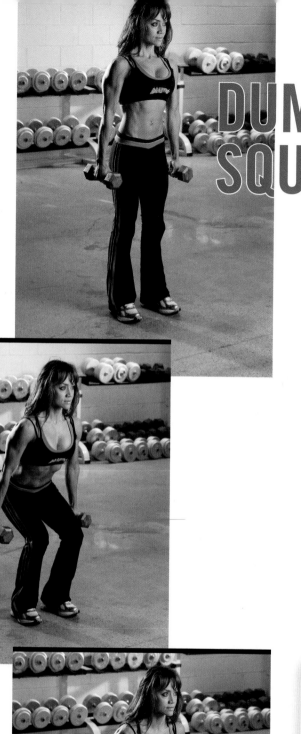

DUMBBELL SQUAT

MUSCLE GROUP: thighs and hips

SETUP:

With your feet shoulder-width apart, stand with dumbbells in each hand, keeping your head up and your chest out.

STEP ONE: Sit back and down as if you were lowering yourself into a chair, letting your upper body bend forward at the hips. If you can, lower yourself until you feel your calves make contact with your hamstrings, making sure not to relax at the bottom of the Squat.

STEP TWO: Push off from your heels to rise from the Squat, making sure not to lean forward or twist.

Tiki Tip: Squats can be difficult to do correctly, so concentrate on keeping the form right and building from there. If you can't squat all the way down at first, just go as far as you can while maintaining form. This is the single best exercise for your thighs and hips.

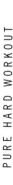

LUNGE

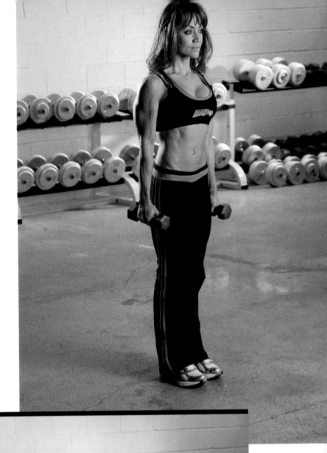

MUSCLE GROUP: thighs, hips, and legs

SETUP:

Hold a pair of dumbbells at your sides.

STEP ONE: From this position, lunge forward with the right foot, transferring all your weight onto that foot and keeping your knee bent at a ninety-degree angle.

STEP TWO: Return to the original position and lunge again, this time with the left foot. Breathe out as you lunge and in as you recover.

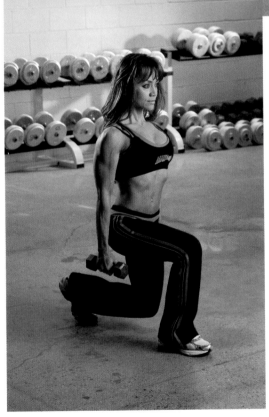

Tiki Tip: Start with light weights, say 5 pounds, and after you get the feel of the movement, you'll be able to add more weight.

LEG SPLITS

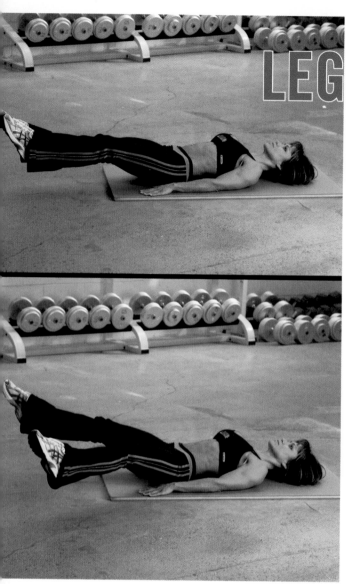

MUSCLE GROUP: inside thigh and abductor muscles

SETUP:

Lie on your back on the floor.

Raise your legs until they are about a foot off the ground.

Move your legs outward until they reach the split position.

STEP ONE: Bring the legs together, still keeping them about a foot off the ground.

STEP TWO: Return to the split position.

Tiki Tip: Adding ankle weights is a good idea as you progress.

SUGGESTED WORKOUT SCHEDULES

This three-days-a-week program for women is a good way to start training if you've had no experience with it before. These eight exercises will give you real results, but of course, you'll have to work at them. Once you've mastered the exercises, you'll want to start challenging yourself with increased repetitions and/or weights.

Squat: 2–3 sets of 12–15 reps

Calf Raise: 2–3 sets of 20–30 reps

Lunge: 2 sets of 12 reps each leg

Leg Raise: 3 sets of as many as possible

Sit-up: 3 sets of as many as possible

Dumbbell Bench Press: 3 sets of 10 reps

Bent-Arm Pullover: 3 sets of 10 reps

Dumbbell One-Arm Row: 3 sets of 10 reps

In addition, women can add a set of one-arm dumbbell stretches or Triceps Dumbbell Kickbacks. Other exercises to consider would be dumbbell biceps curls, and Seated Shoulder Presses.

Below is a four-days-a-week strengthening program for women. Choose among your favorite exercises listed here to build a workout that focuses on areas of your body you particularly wish to work on. For example, if you want to strengthen your triceps and thighs, be sure to include several exercises for those on the appropriate days, and push yourself particularly hard with them. Basically, Mondays and Thursdays you'll be working your lower body; Tuesdays and Fridays you'll be working your upper body. Get in some fun cardio activity on the weekend, whether it's walking, biking, tennis, or whatever.

MONDAY: waist, thighs, and calves

TUESDAY: chest, arms, back, and shoulders

WEDNESDAY: day of rest

THURSDAY: same as Monday

FRIDAY: same as Tuesday

SATURDAY: cardio activity without weights

SUNDAY: cardio activity without weights

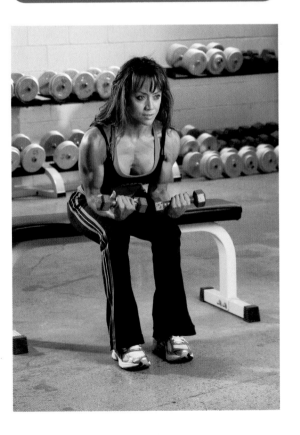

WOMEN AND WEIGHTLIFTING

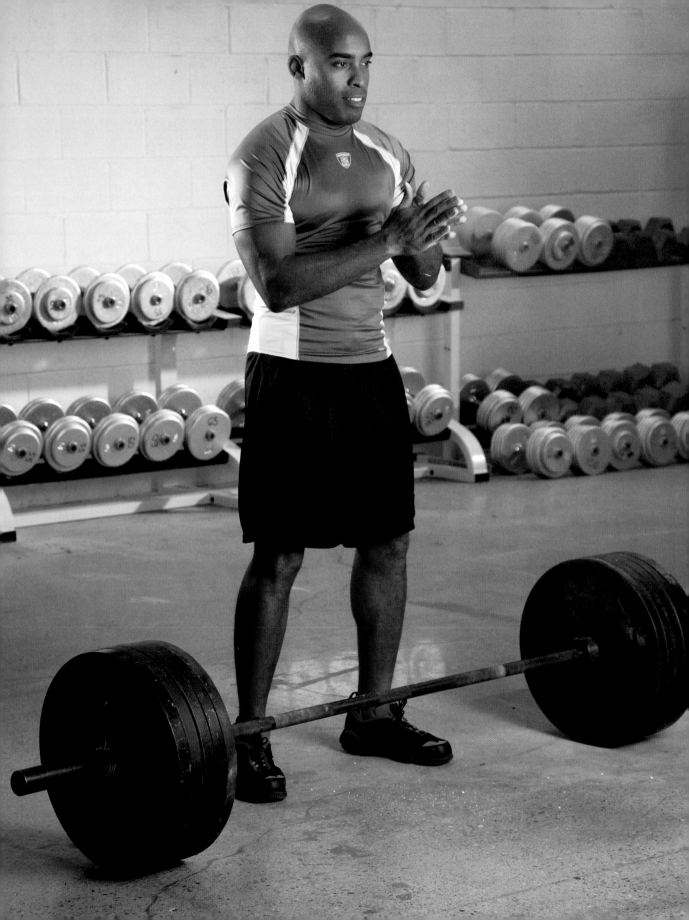

BEYOND SUCCESS AND STAYING MOTIVATED

I think I've always had the right kind of motivations and ideals," Tiki has said. "I think my mother was a great influence with how she raised us, just by her struggles being a single mother with two kids, working numerous jobs, and forcing us to be independent early. We learned the value of hard work, and it's stuck with me in everything I've done, whether it was as high school valedictorian, or going to college and excelling in business school, or becoming a professional athlete.

"It's never been easy for me. I've always been small, always told that I couldn't achieve things. But I've always believed in myself and as my mom always said, 'You believe in yourself, because if you don't, no one else will.' I think that has pushed me."

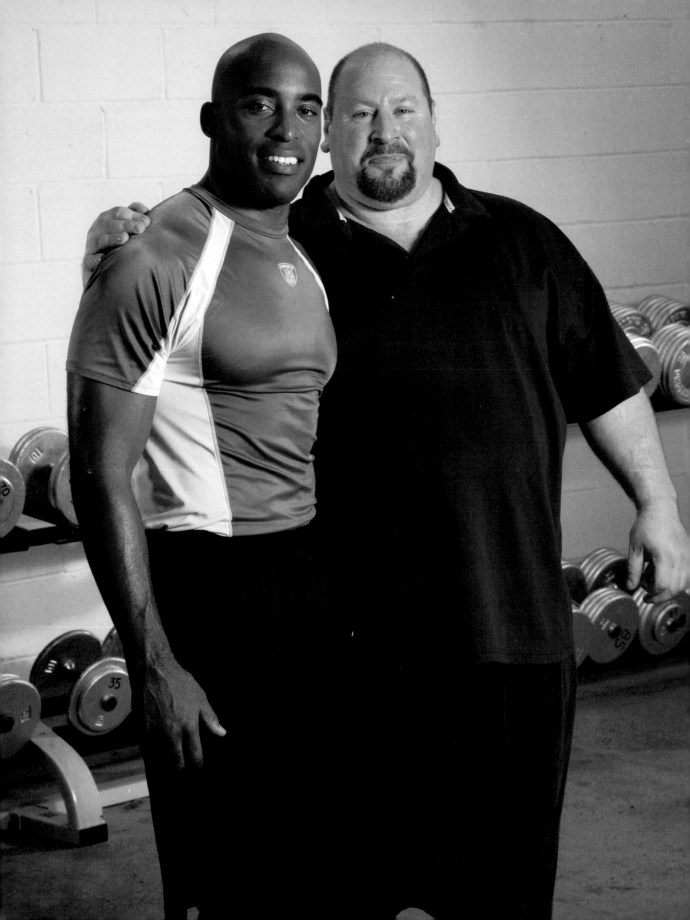

ACKNOWLEDGMENTS

TIKI BARBER: I'd first like to thank my wonderful wife, Ginny, for supporting me in everything I do and for giving me two beautiful sons, A.J. and Chason. Thanks to my mother for teaching me the value of hard work and to Ronde for being by my side all these years. Mark Lepselter has been my close friend and confidant for many years, and I owe him additional thanks for introducing me to Joe. Thanks to all my Giants teammates throughout the years and to the Giants organization for a great decade. Thanks to Scott Waxman and Byrd Leavell at the Waxman Agency, to Scott Hays, and to my editor, Patrick Mulligan, publisher Bill Shinker, and the whole team at Gotham for bringing this book together. And, of course, last but not least, I have to thank the Big Man, Joe Carini, for transforming my body, making me mentally stronger, and preparing me for the best years of my football career.

JOE CARINI: I would like to thank my beautiful wife, Joan Pecchio Carini, for always being by my side. Without her this book would never have been written. To my son, Eric, the Big E. I'm proud of you, Son. I also would like to acknowledge my mom—the inspiration of my life. She taught me the meaning of pure hard work. I love you dearly, Mom. Naturally, this book would never have materialized if I had never had the opportunity to meet Tiki and his brother, Ronde. They trusted me, and believed in my madness. These are great men, and I feel privileged to consider them my friends. We will always keep on; we don't know any other way. Last, I'd like to thank Mark Lepselter—the big believer in all of us. Words cannot describe how grateful I am to Lep. He changed my life by allowing me the privilege of training Tiki and Ronde.

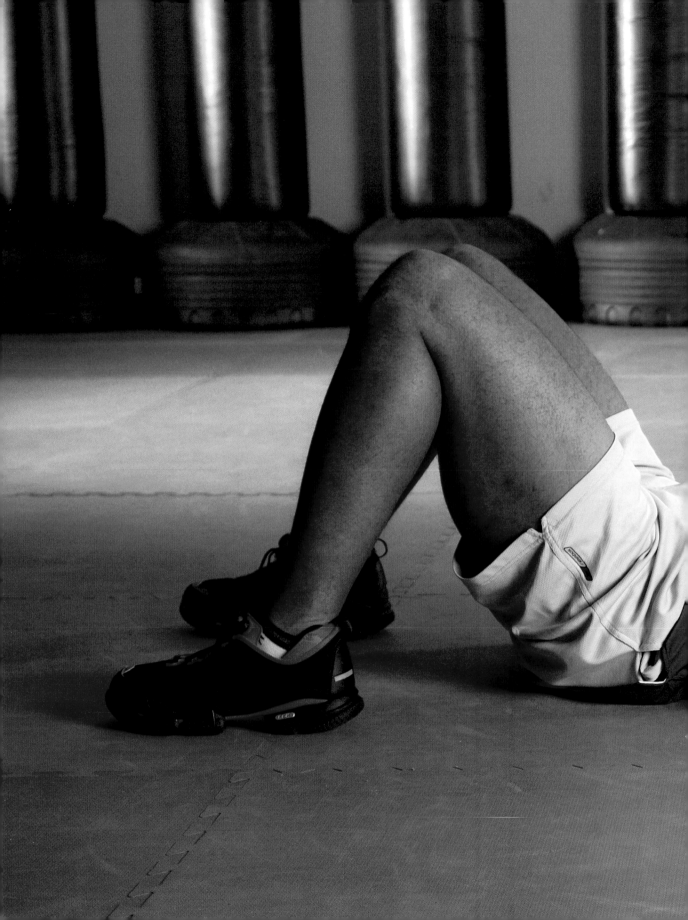

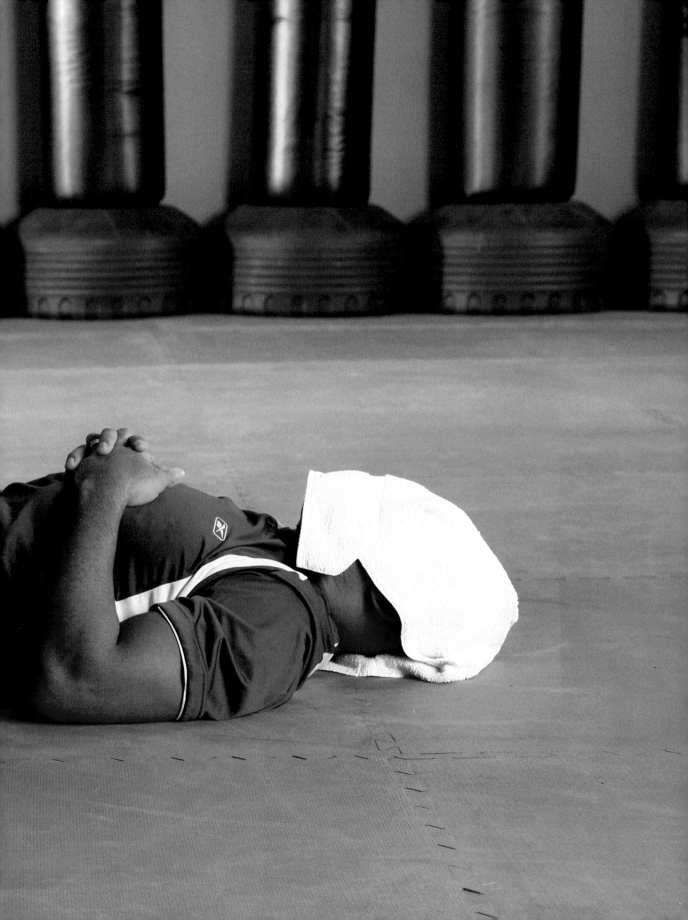

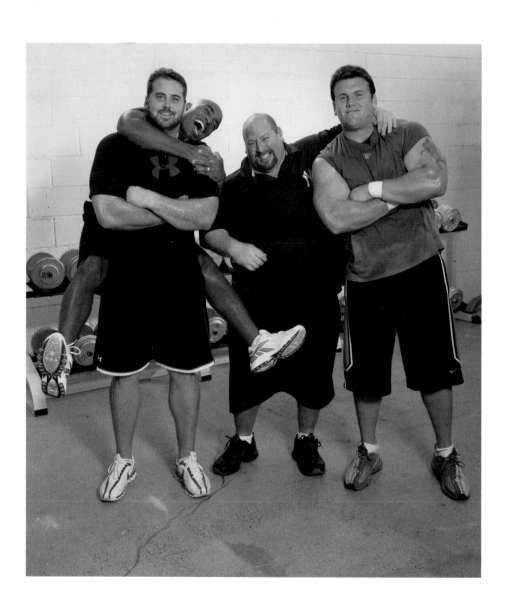